This book is dedicated to my family.

First to my wife, Jen, whom I just adore, and my boys, Kyle and Josh, along with their wives, and of course, to my firstborn grandson, Matthew (aka, Matty Mac, aka Triple M). One day you'll read this, and I want you to know your "PaPa" loves you!

Next, to my community of clients, both near and far. You trusted me to be your trainer and to experiment with you to get the best results.

Finally, to my church family: you always support me. Thank you!

Library Of Congress Cataloging-In-Publication Data

McKinney, Steve. The gospel of fitness: a rational approach to aging gradefully / by Steve McKinney

p. cm.

ISBN 979-8-9922245-0-4 (softcover)

1. Fitness. 2. Exercise. 3. Diet. I. Title.

Edited by Zach Swee

Printing number

FP 23 24 25

7 6 5 4 3 2 1

Praise for *THE GOSPEL OF FITNESS*

"This is a must-read for everyone, not just those seeking to "Age Gracefully." In today's 'go-to-the-internet-for-advice' world, there is a dire need for practical science-based fitness and nutrition information. Steve McKinney's *The Gospel of Fitness* does just that. It covers all relevant topics for those pursuing a prudent approach to the popular goals of losing fat, building muscle, feeling better, and living a long and healthy life. It is comprehensive but easy to understand. It addresses questions regarding current trends and products. It provides pragmatic tips you can apply to your daily routine, debunks myths, and offers practical alternatives. Most importantly, it is safe and healthy. Steve's *Gospel* will save you valuable time and effort with a straightforward path to your goal(s). Apply discipline and effort—two requisites for success at anything—and you are on your way to a long, healthy, and prosperous life."

Tom Kelso, MS, MSCC-E, CSCS, Head Strength and Conditioning Coach, UF, SEMO, & UIC

"It's an honor to endorse *The Gospel of Fitness* by my friend and colleague of over 20 years, Steve McKinney of Fitness And More. Steve's dedication to health and wellness is unparalleled, and this book is a testament to his vast technical knowledge, expertise, and unwavering integrity. His insights and commitment to the science and art of fitness make this book a must-read for anyone serious about transforming their health. His work not only educates but also inspires, and I can confidently say that his influence in the fitness world is as genuine as his friendship has been to me throughout all these years."

Liam Bauer, Strength and Conditioning Coach, Co-owner of TNT Strength

"Steve McKinney is a true servant leader who was put on Earth to help individuals become better versions of themselves—physically, mentally, and spiritually. *The Gospel of Fitness* is a blueprint for living a healthier lifestyle that this world so desperately needs. Steve's entire life has been committed to fitness, and he has helped countless people enhance their lives. This book is a MUST-READ."

Adam Marburger, *President and CEO, Ascent Dealer Services*

"Steve McKinney lays out a proven path to reclaim your health, shed unwanted fat, and build lasting strength. With decades of hands-on experience, Steve is as authentic as they come—a true expert who has dedicated his life to helping clients achieve their full potential. His passion for transforming lives shines through on every page. Read this book. Take it to heart. Follow his guidance—you'll unlock the best version of yourself."

Lawrence Neal, *High Intensity Business*

THE GOSPEL OF FITNESS
A Rational Approach to Aging Gracefully

How to Lose 20 Pounds of Fat in 8 Weeks and Gain Strength

THE
GOSPEL of
FITNESS

A Rational Approach To Aging Gracefully

LOSE UP TO
20
POUNDS

and

GAIN STRENGTH IN
8
WEEKS

STEVE MCKINNEY

FORGE PRESS

FOREWORD

As I tied the belt around his waist, I have to admit I got a little emotional. After all, I have dedicated the majority of my life to martial arts, and this was a huge milestone. Steve McKinney was not only one of my first students, but now he was the first student I had promoted to the level of Black Belt in Brazilian Jiu-Jitsu. This is a major accomplishment that few people in the world achieve. It's a physical and emotional investment that can take between eight to fifteen years. However, I kept it together because this moment was not about me. It was about recognition of Steve's many years of hard work and dedication to the mastery of a very tough, yet rewarding discipline. The more incredible thing is that Steve simultaneously has demonstrated the same level of dedication and passion to helping others through both evangelism and health and fitness.

Steve McKinney is many things to many people. For example, I personally turn to him for wise counsel on several important things. Whether it's with help understanding the bible, advice on a tough decision or frequent guidance on fitness and nutrition, Steve has the answers. While I was a former professional athlete, he helped me maximize my performance at the highest level (fighting in the UFC). And now, as a middle-aged husband, father and entrepreneur, he helps me enhance my health and longevity. In the same way I have dedicated my life to martial arts, Steve has dedicated his life to helping others achieve better health and fitness. In fact, over the years I have personally witnessed dozens of transformations, where he helped clients from all ages and backgrounds become more fit and live healthier, happier lives. These are just a few of the reasons this book from Steve is an incredibly valuable tool for aging with grace and vitality.

In these pages you will not only learn Steve's proven methods from over thirty years in the fitness field. You will also learn how to implement enduring habits that will cultivate a positive lifestyle shift. Empowered with the knowledge in this book we hope you live longer, but more importantly we hope you live better and enjoy life more completely.

Best regards,

Kyle Watson
Owner of Watson Martial Arts, 3rd Degree BJJ
Black Belt, UFC Veteran, The Ultimate Fighter
12 Participant

CONTENTS

INTRODUCTION

Aging Gracefully: A New Perspective

One of my long term clients is a chiropractor. He's been with me for a long time and we talk about the aging process, we talk about injuries, and we talk about the medical options available for those who are starting to notice the decline.

One day we were talking about aging and what more we could do about it and he said this, "We're doing everything we can, we just have to learn to age gracefully." That stuck with me, "Aging gracefully!"

What does it mean to "Age Gracefully?"

Here's my take on aging gracefully. I acknowledge that I'm aging and I look at the latest research on what I can do, what I can control, and then I leave the rest to God. I'm not going to get younger or faster or even stronger but what I can do is simply fight back against the decline of aging.

Aging gracefully is about embracing the process of growing older while maintaining a positive outlook, good health, and a sense of purpose.

It's knowing that I'm getting older but keeping my physical strength for as long as I can. It's keeping my mental health, my spiritual health, and emotional health as priorities in my life.

It's learning to do what I can do and accepting the limits of what I can't do.

It's gracefully enjoying every moment that I can enjoy!

Why I Wrote This Book

Both my parents died at the age of 49.

My mother died on Christmas morning, 1988, in my arms.

Her final words were "Serve Jesus and tell your brother to serve Jesus". I really had no idea of what that meant at the time.

My dad died after a long bout with cancer. It devastated the family. Not just his death, but his dying. Long term care when you're not equipped is more than difficult.

They died too young. They missed so much. They didn't take care of themselves. They simply didn't know any better.

I'm sure you've lost people before their time. It affects everyone.

One of the main reasons I wrote this book is because I want people to live the best quality of life possible—not just for a moment, but for a lifetime. This isn't about a quick fix or a temporary solution; it's about showing you how to build a lasting lifestyle of fitness and well-being and it's also about teaching people to be healthy.

I began my personal training business over 30 years ago, starting in my garage, which I converted into a gym. At first, I charged clients by the month, but soon, they began asking for more personalized plans: "Can you design a workout for me?" "Can you write up a diet plan?" As demand grew, I realized that what people needed most was individual guidance, so I shifted from monthly memberships to one-on-one training.

I also kept records and did observational research. What was working and what wasn't? What can a client sustain over the long haul? Not just a diet plan but a lifestyle change. How can we implement that?

That's where I developed a system of anti-aging fitness. I call it the **"3-W Approach To Fitness."**

Weight training for short sessions, 1-3 times per week, can change your life.

Walking at the right time of day can increase your body's ability to burn fat and it's a great time for prayer or meditation.

Watching your diet by creating an eating lifestyle rather than a diet that will never last.

This system is simple; it's not easy, but it is simple, and simplicity in this day and age is important. What I've done with this system is sorted through all the confusion that people struggle with to help you to learn to "Age Gracefully."

My intention with this book is to change your life! Literally! As a physical trainer and health expert for over 30+ years, I've witnessed true transformation in my clients by following the systems and practices I'll lay out in this book. I truly believe the ideas in this book can change your life and allow you to age gracefully.

PART 1 - THE PROBLEM

The truth is nearly half of Amercians are overweight. [1]

The truth is being overweight causes many problems for us and costs us a lot of money.

Another truth is we want to lose that fat weight and we want to do it now!

We've seen all the information on how we, as Americans, are more overweight than ever. This includes our kids as well. Add the pandemic and we've gained even more weight! We're actually the fattest nation on earth!

Not only that, we're more depressed and hopeless than we've been before. There are many reasons for that as well.

I could explain why we're heading in this direction but I'd rather show you how to get out of it.

There are three reasons we're struggling.

The first reason is what's called:

Disuse atrophy.

What that means is our muscles are atrophying or getting smaller. When your muscles get smaller from not challenging them it, lowers your metabolism, thereby making you susceptible to fat gain.

The Cleveland Clinic, describes it this way: *Disuse (physiologic) atrophy is caused by not using your muscles enough. If you stop using your muscles, your body won't waste the energy it needs to take care of them. Instead, your body will start to break your muscles down, which causes them to decrease in size and strength.* [2]

There are ways to prevent and/or treat this condition.

The best way is through Resistance Strength Training, or to put it simply, lifting weights.

The problem is we don't know what to do, how often to do it, and the proper way to do it efficiently.

Over the years, my favorite ways to combat this problem is what's called "High Intensity Training." I learned this many years ago by reading the work of Arthur Jones, the inventor of Nautilus machines.

The second reason we're struggling is:

We eat too much food.

We also eat too much of the wrong food. We feed our brains rather than our stomachs.

I'll show you some ways for dealing with this problem.

And the third and final struggle is:

We sit around too much.

We go from work to the dinner table to the couch so we can do it all over again the next day.

How do we deal with this problem?

We combine our training with a lifestyle change in the way we eat and then we add a bit of walking to complete the plan.

Warning - it's simple, but it's not easy! The plan requires you to learn some new disciplines that are very doable. You simply have to commit to it. We combine prayer with it as well.

Once you make that commitment, we'll start our six week program that'll hopefully change your life!

That's my goal for you.

Lifestyle change.

But to change is to fight, so let's look at what we're fighting...

What We're Fighting

Fight #1 - Aging

"You can't go back and change the beginning, but you can start where you are and change the ending." - C.S. Lewis

From birth to about 35 years old, we gain physical capabilities. After that, it all slowly begins to change. This is called aging and it happens to everyone.

You don't always notice it but it begins to happen. A loss of strength is mostly unnoticed until you reach down to pick something up and you think, "That felt heavier than before."

But you move on without putting much more thought to it. It compounds little by little from there and one day, you notice everything is not ok. I can't move like I once did. I've gained weight. I'm fighting depression. My joints hurt a bit.

Recently a friend posted something on social media. "I sure wish I felt better." She went to the doctor and was diagnosed with Type 2 diabetes, which, by the way, is treatable with exercise and diet. She was chronically overweight and sedentary.

She then talked about how they were trying to adjust her meds as she was having a reaction to the ones she was given.

She was fine, until she wasn't. She was aging, and it all seemed to hit her at once; even though it was a slow process, she just noticed it one day.

Everything is okay until it isn't.

Here's what's happening:

Muscle mass declines about 10% per decade after age 35. [3]

Life then gets in the way, and we slowly lose our way.

We lose our purpose and just drift from day to day, which eventually leads to helplessness and, in some cases, depression.

The worldwide pandemic made this even more prevalent.

Then we begin to embrace it: "I'm just getting older". And yes, we are getting older every day but a lot of the symptoms we associate with old age–such as weakness, loss of balance, even depression–are symptoms of inactivity, not age.

Simply put, as you age, you lose strength.

If we don't fight back, you will experience a steady physical decline until "old age" renders us frail and helpless. I see this regularly in my training business; people come in to see me and some of them have trouble walking from the car to the gym door.

The good news is, this "age decline" is not inevitable. Many of the diseases associated with aging and frailty are due to loss of muscle.

But we have to do something about it. We can't just accept it; we need to fight back!

How then do we fight back?

We have to know our next enemy to fight and this enemy has a name.

Fight #2 - Sarcopenia - Loss of Muscle as We Age

"I intend to live forever, or die trying." – Gracho Marx

As we age we lose both strength and muscle. It's inevitable but we can slow the process, if we're smart about it.

Sarcopenia [4] is associated with:

- Osteoporosis
- Weakness
- Loss of balance
- Heart disease
- Weight gain
- Type 2 diabetes
- Slow walking speed
- Loss of mobility
- Depression

Isn't it interesting that sarcopenia is associated with depression?

This is aging without fighting back!

We lose strength, we lose purpose, we also decline in our breathing capacity which is associated with weakness.

Aerobic capacity declines about 5% per decade starting at age 30 and 20% per decade after age 70.

By age 70, most Americans have lost 35-40% of the muscle mass and 20% or more of the aerobic capacity they had in their 30s. [5]

I recently had a client start training with me. He wasn't overweight but was getting older and noticing a loss of strength and his breathing was a bit of an issue.

We started building up his strength and slowly his breathing was getting better. When I mean slowly, what I'm saying is it's almost unnoticeable. It's very subtle.

Then he got COVID and everything really went into decline.

When he started back, his breathing was worse than when he started, which prompted him to tell me, "This isn't working."

My reply: "You've been sick, your lungs are struggling to recover, you've lost the strength and progress we've made, and it's going to take some time to get it all back."

I told him he needed to be gracious to his body as it's fighting to regain its baseline before it can build new strength.

My point is, we don't always understand the depth of the battle we fight.

We really are at war with aging. I think it's important that we age gracefully but we don't age without a fight.

We must develop a strategy.

A properly designed strength training program can build and maintain an individual's strength and muscle mass as he/she ages chronologically.

There's a book called *Biomarkers* by William Evens, PhD, and Irwin H. Rosenberg, MD. They are professors of nutrition and medicine at Tufts University. The book identifies 10 "biomarkers" that we can control. [6] Here they are:

- Muscle Mass
- Strength
- Basal Metabolic Rate
- Body Fat Percentage
- Aerobic Capacity
- Blood-Sugar Tolerance
- Cholesterol/HDL Ratio
- Blood Pressure
- Bone Density
- Ability to Regulate Internal Temperature

Here's what's beautiful:

All 10 biomarkers can be improved with a focused strength training program.

Fight #3 - Fat Gain

"It's getting harder and harder to breathe."– Maroon 5

I was listening to the radio while driving yesterday. The radio host was talking about how much exercise it takes to counter the effects of the candy we eat at halloween.

I looked it up and came across this from *Family Food*: [7]

- A snack-size Reese's Cup (1 piece) contains 90 calories and would require 10 minutes of jogging to burn off.

- A fun-size Snickers bar (1 piece) contains 80 calories and would require 9 minutes of jogging to burn off.

- A regular-size Twizzlers Twist Strawberry candy (1 piece) contains 40 calories and would require 5 minutes of jogging to burn off.

- A fun-size Twix bar contains 125 not-so-fun-sized calories, which requires 14 minutes of jogging to burn off.

- A small handful of candy corn (about 20 pieces) contains around 150 calories, in which you would need to carve out 17 minutes for a jog to burn it off.

If you think about it, you rarely, if ever, eat just one piece. Remember the old Lay's Potato Chip catchphrase: "Bet you can't eat just one"?

On a daily basis, an average 160-pound man needs around 2,000 calories to maintain his weight if he's moderately active. A woman who weighs 140 pounds needs about 1,400-1,500 calories. According to Wellfit.com, the average American eats 3,600 calories per day.

My experience with weight gain has been interesting. I've noticed over the years that if I gain about 5 pounds—and this happens sometimes in the cold winter months—I will get in my car, put the seatbelt on, and notice I actually have trouble taking a deep breath.

It really does get harder and harder to breathe.

The reason we gain weight is because we eat too many calories. It's that simple.

I've heard experts say calories don't matter. I couldn't disagree more. Calories do matter and they matter a lot.

Fight # 4 - Loss of Balance

"I'm losing my balance more and more." – Multiple Personal Training Clients

I don't know if you remember the commercial, "I've fallen, and I can't get up." It was a commercial for a product to alert people that you're in a dangerous situation. I'm not in any way making light of that particular situation, but in some cases, there's a chance at making sure that doesn't happen.

One of my chiropractic clients referred his dad to me.

On the initial visit, one of his concerns was the loss of balance as he aged.

"You're most likely losing strength, which affects your balance."

He looked at me in disbelief. I could see it in his face.

A few weeks later, he brought in a newspaper clipping. (By the way, a newspaper is a way we used to get information.)

The clipping was from a question-and-answer forum called, "Ask the Doctor."

He was excited to show me what it said.

"Steve, you were right! Look at this. The Ask the Doctor guy said the same thing you did about my balance and my strength: I'm losing my balance because I'm losing my strength."

Generally, that's the case.

As we get older we slowly lose the balance we had. [8] And you don't have to be "old" to notice this. For some people, it starts early.

I know for me personally, I notice it when I train jiu-jitsu. It's not a huge decline, but I can just tell I'm not as balanced as I used to be.

I'm working with a client who has had multiple surgeries and she's really struggling with balance and walking. We are simply training her for strength. I'm not sure if we can reverse the loss of balance, but I do know we can delay it.

As a side note, she's been through physical therapy, but to no avail. So we're experimenting with different strength training protocols to improve her condition as best we can.

There are multiple reasons for the loss of balance, including side effects from medication, inner ear issues, fatigue, etc. So we need to have a proper diagnosis when we move forward.

Once we have that diagnosis, we'll need the treatment, and there are a lot of treatments out there.

For example, there's the 'stand on one leg' exercise for balance. And this works—if you want to stand on one leg.

I'll explain.

There's something called the S.A.I.D. principle. The NFPT defines it this way in a March 13, 2013 blog: [9] *"The SAID principle says **every sport poses its own unique demands and that in order to improve skills unique to a particular sport, it's best to practice the moves used in that sport.** SAID is the acronym for Specific Adaptation to Imposed Demands."*

Here's how it applies to balance practices:

If I practice standing on one leg, do you know what I'll be good at? You got it! Standing on one leg. You can apply this to most any practice.

The reason it's used to help with balance is the client is generally weak from loss of strength and almost any practice will help improve strength slightly, which will help with the balance issue.

My thought is to increase strength with a safe program and then practice not only walking, but learning how to get up from the floor.

Fight # 5 - Loss of Hope

"I do not account my life of any value nor as precious to myself, if only I may finish my course and the ministry that I received from the Lord Jesus, to testify to the gospel of the grace of God."
– The Apostle Paul

The last part of the decline is a mental/spiritual one. *I was at a wedding recently and I was having a conversation with a young man and he was trying to explain the struggle he was dealing with but was having trouble putting words to it. I listened and then realized what he was saying. Finally, I said, "John, you've lost your hope; you're dealing with hopelessness." It was like a light bulb went on. "Yeah, that's it! That's what I'm dealing with."*

We lose our purpose in life, we lose our identity, and **we lose our hope.**

Hope is the life force that keeps us going and gives us something to live for.

Hope is crucial in dealing with life's problems and maintaining resilience in the face of obstacles.

Even a glimmer of hope that our situation will turn around can keep us going.

The loss of hope happens in many ways.

Illness, the loss of friends and family, job stresses, financial issues, interpersonal conflict, and on it goes.

This is death by a thousand paper cuts.

It's not just one big event (although it can be), it's the daily dings that steal our joy.

It subtly chips away at us and then the next thing you know…

You're existing rather than living.

Earlier in the year of 2022, I had a run of officiating eight funerals. It was unusual to do that many, but I went from funeral to preaching without any time off. One right after the next and at the time, my thought was, "I have to do these and then I have to preach."

The odd thing was, they weren't stopping. I'd get through one and then I'd get a call for another.

Add the normal, everyday issues of life, and I noticed I was struggling with the day-in, day-out of everyday life. It was what I call "the dark night of the soul."

I finally decided, at the urging of my wife, to take some time away and really focus on what I'm called to do, which is both my fitness business and pastoring my church.

I found a book called Resilient by an author I really like, John Eldredge. He had an app that went along with the book, and I used that app daily—actually twice a day.

As I prayed through it, there was a particular day when I made a simple request: "Jesus, enter into this darkness I'm feeling and show me what's going on."

A few hours later, I was near my kitchen table when I had what I call an unintentional thought: "Karen."

Karen was one of the funerals I officiated. She and her husband were the first people I met after I gave my life to the Lord. They were in our first home Bible study, and we all became friends.

I was realizing that I hadn't properly grieved the loss of my friends.

Out of those eight funerals, five were people I talked to on a regular basis—people I had coffee with, shared stories with, and saw on a weekly basis.

I did a total reset and began to dig deeper into what I was dealing with. I noticed I was slowly getting better and thinking more clearly.

As we get older—and by that, I mean every decade—things change, and we have to recognize that and adapt.

What I was able to do when I was 40 is not what I was able to do at 50, and as I hit 60, I wasn't able to do what I could at 50. You get the picture.

I am slowly reminding myself of that. I'm thinking a bit differently about rest and recovery. I'm choosing to engage in relationships that are life-giving, not battery-draining. I'm no longer pushing myself to the limit day in and day out.

As I do, I'm going from hopelessness to hopefulness.

Hope is looking to enjoy what you do and live your passion.

Here's a simple way to get your hope back—ask yourself this:

What do I love to do?

What would I do if money weren't an issue? For me, I love training clients. I love writing about fitness. I love doing public speaking on fitness. I love training jiu-jitsu. I love preaching the Gospel. I love hanging out with my wife, kids, and grandkids. I love helping people live a better life, hence my purpose is to teach people how to "Age Gracefully."

Give your life some meaning by making life better for others and for yourself!

Bill Pearl was a bodybuilding legend, and he said the best guidance he ever got was from his father, who told him to accomplish at least one positive thing every day, even if it was just cutting the grass.

Meaningful work gives life purpose.

Mistakes That Add To The Problem

I have a library of books on strength and fitness. I've studied and experimented with what to do and what not to do. I've made progress, but I've also made mistakes. I've injured myself by training too heavy, incorrectly planning, using poor form, not getting proper feedback, and not understanding how your body works.

But, I've learned, and I've learned a lot. I've learned through mistakes, through trial and error, and through conferring with experts who knew more than I. I've learned the key components to exercise.

There are three key components to any fitness program.[10] They are muscular strength, aerobic capacity, and flexibility. My system hits all three.

Muscular strength is built through progressive resistance exercise or weight training. Aerobic capacity is also built by reducing rest time betweens sets, which keeps your heart rate elevated. Flexibility is developed by training your muscles through a full range of motion.

Understanding those three keys are the best way to build a foundation of health and wellness.

One of the questions I ask a client when they come in for an initial visit with me is, "What have you tried before to get in shape, and how did it work for you?" I tracked the answers and identified ten common mistakes people make when trying to regain their health.

These mistakes really cause a lot of problems because we put so much effort into getting where we want to be it exhausts us and we end up just spinning our wheels, and eventually, we get discouraged and give up.

Here are the ten mistakes we make:

Mistake #1 – Going In Like a Lion And Out Like a Lamb

Happy New Year! Don't forget to make resolutions you won't keep and put up a wall calendar you won't look at!

I'm going to start an exercise program on Monday (it always starts on Monday, for some reason). I'm going to exercise five days per week for an hour a day and I'm going to completely change my diet and eat nothing but super nutritious food and I'm going to quit smoking and drinking.

How's that working out?

Diets are short term; lifestyle changes are long term. My goal for you is to make a lifestyle change that will last. To do that we have to approach the program with a plan. The plan will start very narrow and then it will get more broad.

We will start with a diet plan. I'll suggest what to eat and when to eat. We'll do that for eight weeks. During that time, you'll begin to understand how your body reacts to certain exercises, foods, etc. You'll also learn what you can do and what you can't. You'll get a picture of a normal week and you'll adjust accordingly.

You'll 'fall off the wagon' at times, but knowing that will allow you to get right back on it.

Here's a story about Jeff and his first visit with me:

Jeff walked through my door for his first visit. "Jeff, how are you?" I asked.

"I'm good, but I've gained a bunch of weight and lost my motivation. That's why I'm here."

"Ok, I got it," I responded. "Tell me, Jeff, have you worked out before?"

"I sure have," Jeff responded. "I was in great shape. I worked out for an hour every morning, five days per week, and I lost over 30 pounds. I did that for 2–3 straight months."

"That's really great! Why did you stop?" I asked.

THE GOSPEL OF FITNESS

"I'm not exactly sure. I have a family, and life got really busy. I just couldn't make it to the gym as much, and the diet got a bit monotonous. I guess I really need some help getting back into it," was his response.

"Ok, Jeff, I want you to think about something. Training five days per week for an hour adds up to a lot of time. When you factor in the commute to and from the gym, you're probably up to an hour and a half. That's 7 ½ hours per week. Multiply that by four, and you're up to 30 hours per month. Jeff, that's like adding a part-time job to your life, and it's not sustainable. Does that make sense to you?" I asked.

"It sure does," Jeff replied.

"Here's what I want to do. I'm going to set a goal for you. We're going to drop 20 pounds of fat, and we're going to keep your strength up while we do it. You're going to train two days per week, do a little walking, and start counting calories. This will give you a great foundation, and we'll build some habits of health and longevity that you can use for the rest of your life. You're going to take it slow and treat your body well. It'll take the full eight weeks, but it'll work. You good with that?"

"I'm in," Jeff responded.

One of the biggest frustrations for most people is the lack of patience and not looking at health and fitness from the perspective of playing the long game.

Losing fat and gaining muscle takes time. Lots of time. You can't force it to happen, you almost have to coax it to happen.

Mistake #2 - Lack of Direction

"If you can't convince them, confuse them." - Harry S. Truman

Flipping tires, running miles, jumping on boxes, dragging sleds—
and on it goes. Keto diets, vegan diets, carnivore diets—and
on it goes. Taking vitamins, drinking concoctions, seven-day
cleanses—and on it goes.

Here's the reality.

There's an overload of information. And it's very very confusing.

Do you want to know why?

There's money to be made. [11]

If you have any idea what's going on Instagram, TikTok, Facebook,
or any social media platform, there are a lot of influencers. There's
money to be made as long as you have content. It doesn't always
have to be true or safe; you just need to put out content.

In my fitness business, I get clients who come in for a consultation. One of my questions to kick off our conversation is, "Do you
have any goals?" I get a lot of different answers. "I need to work
on my core." "I just want to feel better." "I need to lose weight."

Because I've been at this for a while, I generally help them set
their goals. Most people I deal with have gained fat, declined in
aerobic capacity, and lost strength. We then sit down, I explain

how to deal with that and I simply show them what's happened. For the most part, they understand it. I also like to ask, "When did you start noticing this change?"

"I don't really know exactly, but it seems like it happened overnight."

I then begin to explain, using my system, how to start making the change to get back to feeling better. It reduces the confusion by reducing complexity. Too much information causes what's called information overload.

People need simple direction!

According to RescueTime.com: "Information overload occurs when a person is exposed to more information than the brain can process at one time." As we take in more and more complex information in less time and have more options laid out in front of us, our brains panic and freeze.

Simple is always better as long as the simple that you're putting into practice is true.

Mistake #3 - Not Having Goals

"Never quit. It is the easiest cop-out in the world. Set a goal and don't quit until you attain it. When you do attain it, set another goal, and don't quit until you reach it. Never quit." –Bear Bryant

When I talk about "goals," I'm simply talking about: what is the reason you want to get in shape?

What's the reason you want to lose fat and get strong again? You really want to know your goals, as it'll keep you going when all the emotion wears off.

Here's an example:

As I said earlier, both my parents died at a young age. The other part of that was my dad lived a major portion of his life with illness and depression. He lost his job, and when he did, he lost his identity. Looking back, it was rather sad.

I think on a personal level that's a big motivator for me.

*I really do practice what I preach and I want to **"Age Gracefully."** That's not just a cliché.*

My goal is to **"Age Gracefully"** so that I can enjoy my family and continue with my purpose of helping others do the same.

This is a quote from the National Library of Medicine: "Goal setting is an important element in physical activity (PA) and dietary interventions. Goal-setting techniques are effective in helping individuals initiate and maintain health behavior over time."

We want to develop a lifestyle of healthy habits that will help you keep your weight in a healthy range for as long as possible. This is why we aim to develop a lifestyle of fitness, not just a short-term diet that you go on and then go off. [12]

Goals are important. They relate to your why.

Goals need to be defined.

About 30 years ago, when I started my fitness business, I had a new client come in for his consultation. I asked him what his goals were. He was very specific. "I want to be able to play with my grandchildren." Here's what's awesome to me: he now has grandchildren. He can now play with his grandchildren and he's still an active client!

Goals need to be specific.

'I want to lose weight' is not a specific goal. It's general. It's vague. Reframing the goal to 'I want to lose 20 pounds' is very specific. To be even more specific, you want to put a time frame on it: 'I want to lose 20 pounds in 8 weeks,' which is even more specific. 'I want to lose 20 pounds in 8 weeks and keep it off for the rest of my life!'

Now, my goal got very specific and it went from a short-term goal (8 weeks) to a long-term one: the rest of my life.

Goals need to be reasonable.

'I want to lose 20 pounds in a week.' It isn't reasonable, nor is it healthy. Fat loss goals are usually unreasonable in that we want the fat off and we want it off now.

I've had clients who go on super restrictive diet plans and lose weight only to put it right back on and in some cases even more than before.

Goals can vary.

About a year ago, I had a goal I wanted to reach. I wanted to be able to sprint. I am not a runner, in that I don't jog for fitness as I think that's very hard on your musculoskeletal system. What I mean is, it beats on your joints. I'm not saying it's necessarily bad for you, but what I've seen over the years is runners get addicted to the runners high, which makes them want to run more, and eventually, they end up over training.

Sprinting for some reason is different. It's shorter and doesn't cause as much repetitive response.

One of the reasons/goals I wanted from sprinting was holding onto whatever athleticism I had remaining. I still train Jiu-Jitsu on a regular basis and I assumed—correctly, I might add—that sprinting would help me athletically.

Here's how I approached my goal:

I would do my normal weight training and then once per week, I would try to run sprints right after I trained.

When I started, the only thing I worried about was my stride. I needed to lengthen my stride as over the years my stride was non-existent.

Have you ever seen an old man shuffle with very short strides? I did not want that to happen, if I could avoid it.

I would run five or so sprints based on how I felt—nothing overly taxing, but pushing myself just a bit more each time.

That lasted a few weeks, then I decided that my stride was actually getting better, so then I decided to try to sprint a bit harder. I didn't sprint as hard as I could, as I knew that would cause injury, such as muscle strains and such.

I simply would go out and on the first sprint, I was still working on my stride. On the second sprint, I would still work on my stride but try to lengthen it more. By the third sprint, I would focus on going just a bit faster.

My fourth and fifth sprints would be as hard as I dared—meaning, to sprint as hard as I could without risking injury.

Here I am a year later and I can proudly say I can run a sprint. I still do the same escalation protocol and I still haven't run as fast as I can, but I can run again!

I love doing that. Setting goals and reaching them.

Do I always reach my goals?

Nope.

Do I keep setting goals?

Yep.

Goals are good!

What are your goals? I'm hoping you're wanting to lose 20 pounds in 8 weeks!

Mistake #4 – Relying on Technology

I had a client come to me one day, and he was near tears. He was a grown man. (I always joke about how the scale can bring a grown man to tears.)

"I'm not losing weight." "Tell me how much you're eating." "I'm eating 2,200 calories per day."

"You're eating too much," I said. He aggressively pointed to his Fitbit. "But my Fitbit is telling me I can eat that much."

"Your Fitbit is wrong!" [13]

This person was measuring activity and adding calories because of said activity and then doing more to eat more. I'm not a fan of Fitbits. Actually, there's nothing wrong with them, but they don't work for me. Here's why:

Too much data confuses me. It's just how my mind works (or doesn't work).

I get overwhelmed easily, so tracking too much hinders me, rather than helps me.

You might be different in that you like the feedback. I say if that much data works for you, then use it, but I always think simple is better.

Here's an example.

I had a client years ago who came to me to get stronger and lose fat. I designed the program, but the client was obsessed with the number of steps they took per day. They did up to 20,000 steps on certain days, but never less than 10,000, unless a sickness came about.

When the client would come in, they would always want to show me how many steps they did yesterday, to which I would respond, "That's great, now let's step on the scale."

There was no movement on the scale, and in some cases, there was an actual weight gain.

Why does this happen?

There are a few reasons. The first one is that excessive exercise can increase certain hormones in your body.

Endocrine Web reports, "If you like to go hard with HIIT, just beware of overdoing it, which can have the opposite effect on your hormones, leading to excess adrenaline and cortisol. Overexercsing can increase our stress hormones, and raise the risk of muscle loss, injury, and fatigue."

Here's what else is interesting: when you have that increase in hormonal response, the easiest way to feel better is to eat.

Generally the food most used to 'put out the hormonal fire' is simple carbohydrates, which can lead to excess weight gain.

I recently saw this in a client who was training for a marathon. This client actually gained weight from the extra running, as it caused them to over eat.

It can be so confusing.

What then do we do?

We measure!

Let's talk about what we measure.

Mistake # 5 - Not Measuring

"If you can't measure it, you can't improve it." - Peter Drucker

What do we measure?

What you measure will be based on your goals.

"I'm not losing weight, I'm losing inches" can only go so far if fat loss is your goal.

There's a point where the scale will have to move in the direction you want it to go.

Approximately 90%+ of my clients come to me with these goals:

- **Fat loss**
- **Strength Gain**
- **Feel better**

Fat loss and strength gain are very objective and measurable.

Feeling better is subjective but it does relate to fat loss and strength gain as well.

If fat loss and strength gain are the goals, then you simply need to measure how much weight you're lifting in good form.

Strength is finite, so there's a ceiling to how strong you can get, but the goal is to get as strong as possible and stay strong as long as you can.

The other measurement pertains to fat loss. The scale will determine how you're doing here. It will tell you if you're losing fat or not.

You want to lose fat, not weight. Losing weight includes losing muscle and fat. We want to diminish muscle loss and increase fat loss.

If your strength levels remain good, you'll maintain muscle as you lose weight, as there is somewhat of a correlation between how much weight you can lift in good form and how much muscle you have. It's not exact but it is close.

With that said, here's what we measure (the first two are most important):

- **How much fat am I losing?** We measure this by using the scale.
- **How much strength am I gaining?** We measure this by keeping track of how much I can lift in good form.
- **How are my clothes fitting?** This is a simple objective measurement by checking my clothes.
- **How do I feel?** This is subjective but you should start feeling better.
- **What does my annual blood work reveal?** This is very important to track.

Mistake #6 - Being Too Rigid

"A girl invited me to come out to a Bible study, and I said, 'Why not? I don't have anything to lose.' I went, and to my surprise, I saw people that loved God, but they were not square or rigid. They were just people like me." – American rapper Lecrae

When you start your program, I want you to be all in. I want you to be rigid. You need to do that so we can create a baseline. Once you get the baseline, you can then learn how to create a lifestyle that fits you!

For example, if you need to lose fat, then stay very strict on your diet for the first six weeks or so.

Then you can slowly learn how your body works.

"I feel better when I eat certain foods."

"I feel better when I eat at certain times."

"I feel better when I get a certain amount of sleep."

Those are all great things to learn.

Now, let's set a scenario:

You've been making some changes, you're working out, you're watching what you eat, and you're feeling great. But you have this 'thing' you have to go to. An event. They're going to be serving food and just the thought of that creates a bit of anxiety in you.

How do you handle it? Let me tell you how not to handle it:

Years ago, I was a competitive bodybuilder and we had a family Thanksgiving dinner to attend.

I'm embarrassed to say this but I brought my own food.

Don't go to that extreme. Here's a way to handle it:

You can do a little intermittent fasting (I'll show you what I.F. is in the Watch Your Diet section). Then when you show up you can enjoy the food with everyone else.

And there's a chance you might overeat or over drink. Just go with it and the next day get back on the wagon. The next day might be good for your I.F. as well. Learn to be adaptable. It makes life better.

Recently I was working with a client and explaining to him what is possible if he applies what I taught him. I also explained to him that I' was going to give him an outline. "You need to make that outline fit you. Don't try to fit you into the outline."

What I meant was, "don't set yourself up for failure by making goals that are unreachable. It's like forcing a square peg into a round hole. If you're not an early riser, don't schedule appointments early."

He starts the program. Two weeks later, he quit the program. I asked why and he said it just didn't work for him. As I dug deeper, I found out the foods he was eating weren't agreeing with him.

"Why didn't you just ask me? This is such an easy fix. All you had to do was make some slight adjustments."

My point:

Experiment. Learn how your body works. Adjust.

It's the difference between a rigid plan and a flexible one. Be flexible.

Mistake #7 - Not Having a Routine

"You'll never change your life until you change something you do daily. The secret of your success is found in your daily routine."
– John Maxwell

My son Josh has a Jiu-Jitsu podcast called the 'I Suck At Jiu-Jitsu Show'. In a recent episode, he was talking about how I'm always asking people about their workouts and training—always keeping the team accountable.

That's very true.

The secret of your success is in your daily routine!

I've been preaching that as long as I can remember.

Here's a typical day for me:

Up early, around five-ish. Boil water for my Chemex pour-over coffee.

Turn on my daily prayer app.

Use the bathroom and finish making the coffee.

Listen to the Bible and journal my prayers.

Spend the first few hours studying for sermons.

Based on the day, I'll go workout, train clients, or teach a class.

Come home and break my fast with a protein smoothie. Have dinner. Make sure I walk for 30 minutes or as close to it as I can. Walk with my wife, Jen, if we can coordinate schedules.

Get to bed early. I mean really early, between 7:30-8:00 pm.

Things change but for the most part, that's how I do it.

Do you have a daily routine?

If you don't, is it possible to make small changes to have one? Small changes over time can make the routine work well!

Mistake #8 - Lack of Preparation

"The heart of man plans his way, but the Lord establishes his steps." - Solomon

This is a double-edged sword.

I was catching up with a client I hadn't seen in a while, as she had been working with one of the trainers on my team. Curious to hear her thoughts, I asked how she was enjoying the workouts. She said she loved them. I then asked how her diet was going and she said it went well for about three weeks as she was prepping food, but she had a family and things just got in the way.

This is common but also important to understand.

Food prepping can become a part-time job!

If you do have a family and you try to prepare food for yourself and then different food for your family, that'll only last for a while before you get overwhelmed.

There are ways to handle it: simply prepare foods that are healthy for both you and your family.

But there's also the 'I hate this food, Mom' complaints that go on.

Just slowly introduce new foods to them and at the same time eat with them, but control your food amounts.

Here's the other edge to the sword, this is how it works for me or against me personally:

I really need to know what I'm going to eat that day and I'd like to know early.

Here's why:

I generally eat within a small window of time. It just works for me.

If I don't know what I'm going to eat, I have a tendency to just go with what's quick and easy as I'm not a great cook.

I've remedied that by having some 'go-to's' for healthy food places.

I heard this quote from someone on sermon preparation, but I think it'll fit with meal planning as well:

"As long as the furniture is in the room, you can rearrange it endlessly. But if you are still moving furniture on Saturday night, you're in trouble."

Mistake #9 – Not Prioritizing Your Health

"So many people spend their health gaining wealth, and then have to spend their wealth to regain their health."

When I have a personal training client come in for their initial visit, there's a point where I'll tell them, **"Treat your workouts as doctor's appointments; if you do, you'll have fewer doctor's appointments."**

I really believe that.

Learn to look for reasons to work out, not for reasons not too.

Abbott.com: *Take control of your health by choosing a healthy lifestyle. Eating a healthy diet and getting regular exercise can help you keep your weight, blood sugar level, blood pressure, and cholesterol level in a healthy range.* [14]

What does it look like when I choose to prioritize my health?

There are four pillars of health, or as I like to put it, Anti-Aging. These are from a Dr. Peter Attia podcast called "The Peter Attia Drive" that I listened to a long time ago and it stuck with me:

- **Strength Training**
- **Sleep**
- **Having a spiritual life**
- **Calorie reduction with optimal nutrition**

As I've said before, this really is simple. But it's not always easy.

For me strength training is easy; it's a joy. Sleep is a struggle and I try to navigate it the best I can. As far as calorie restriction, I'm pretty good there as I have a sense of how much food to eat, and I use my walks and such for my spiritual life.

It does take some time to narrow it down but it's very doable.

I recently had a conversation with a client who was diagnosed with a health condition. I told him his condition was controllable IF he would take responsibility and prioritize his health over his wealth. I told him, you can buy a lot of things but health can't be bought, it must be earned!

Mistake #10 - Listening to the Wrong Experts

"Good advice is often annoying; bad advice never is."
– French proverb

This is my final mistake on the list.

As I stated earlier, there's just so much information, it causes a lot of confusion.

I was just talking last week with a friend who had his hip replaced. I was asking him about his therapy. He said he'd been to several therapists and each one had a different twist on how to rehab him.

He told me the most recent one wanted him to learn how to walk differently. I'm thinking, 'you've been walking the same for 40 years or so, changing your walk won't help your hip at this point. Why not just rehab the hip?'

I had another client whose grandson had ruptured a disc in his lower back during high school workouts. The coach just put a program out there and he was doing it and now his back is a total mess and it'll affect him, most likely, for the rest of his life.

I've had countless clients referred to me from chiros and physicians after going through treatment for injuries related to fitness practices that are outright dangerous.

I recently had a client who was coming to me but was also doing a program that involved throwing things and flipping tires. She was 70 years old! I had to tell her I really didn't want to train her as it was inevitable she was going to get injured and unfortunately she did.

The problem in the fitness industry is there's no regulation. I understand that as it's nearly impossible to regulate. Add to that social media and it's a recipe for disaster.

I just saw a post from a guy I know. He's been in the gym for a few weeks. Now he's taking selfies and shaming people for not being in the gym. As people reply to him, he's now telling them he can help them.

Nothing wrong with trying to help people at all, but only if you have the qualifications to do so.

As in any field, there are good trainers and not so good.

Here's how the fitness industry works:

'I like to lift weights. I think I'll be a trainer. Come train with me.'

I love to joke about the same things that happen with people who like to drink and then they want to open a bar.

There's a lot of responsibility in training clients. Just because a person is in shape doesn't mean they know how to train others.

I remember someone saying this, **"If you want to learn how to lift weights, go to the gym and do the opposite of what everyone else is doing."**

I think there's some truth to that.

Are You Willing To Learn?

*"If you are not willing to learn, no one can help you.
If you are determined to learn, no one can stop you."*
- Zig Ziglar

This book is all about learning.

What I've learned about fitness after I thought I knew it all.

What I've learned about getting older, after I thought I knew what it would be like to get older.

What I've learned about the connection between our spiritual and mental health and how it affects our physical health.

I've put this book together as a learning tool but I structured it as a life of learning by using my personal experience, stories, and facts about training and observing clients over many many years.

I've been training clients for over 30 years.

I've been working with people in a church setting for over 20 years.

I'm still learning.

I've heard it said, "When you stop learning, you stop growing." That's just so true!

To learn is to grow.

I'll teach you what I've learned. It's going to be interesting and fun!

Every year, we take a family vacation. Here was my plan: I would diet before vacation and then put it all back on at vacation and then struggle again when I got back from vacation because I didn't have vacation as a goal. It was the whole yo-yo approach to dieting.

A 10-12-pound gain in a week was normal! So was the visit to the ice cream place after dinner every night, followed by the complaints of being, "So full I can't breath."

I had to work hard on making some changes as this way of approaching.

I worked very hard on changing my thinking.

One of the biggest shifts in my thinking happened many years ago. We take yearly vacations to Destin, Florida. (Once I find a place I like, I stick with it.)

On those vacations, I like to learn and read and study. One particular vacation really refined my learning process. I found a website by Dr. Ellington Darden. In this book, he explained his methods and how he approached training clients. I took that website and bought a few of his books and studied. It made sense. I continued to research different methods while I was away.

When I got back from that vacation, I put some ideas to the test. I developed my own system, based on training my clients and testing their results.

I noticed some very dramatic changes in some of my clients and not so dramatic in others.

I found that people who "took ownership" of their health and fitness got the best results.

I found people who prayed did well physically and emotionally.

I discovered ways to simplify fitness and create lifestyle principles rather than programs.

The most important discovery was coming up with plans that people can do for the rest of their lives.

That's what I want to teach you in this book.

I'm going to show you:

- **The basics of exercise.**
- **How to master the basics of exercise.**
- **How you can regain some of your youth by increasing your strength.**
- **A simple eating concept that you can use no matter where you go.**
- **A metabolism hack to burn more fat.**
- **How hormones affect hunger and what to do about it.**

Let's look further.

PART 2 - THE PLAN

My 3-W Approach to Fitness

Years ago, I developed a "System of Fitness." This system applies to everyone, but it does have to be tailored to fit you. You take the program from what I call "general" and make it "specific."

Think of it this way:

You go to find a suit or a dress. When you go, they have what you like. You look for it in your size, but when you find it, you also realize it needs to be tailored to fit you. They tuck a little here and tweak a little there, and before you know it, you find what fits.

As time goes on, your body changes, and the suit or dress you bought has to be altered even further.

The point is to make the program fit you.

Now, let's overview the program.

When I speak at events, I have my audience hold up 3 fingers. What you'll notice, with a little creativity, is that it forms a bit of a "W." That's an easy way to remember the system.

- **The first W in the system is Weight training.**
- **The second W is Watching your diet.**
- **The third W is Walking or some form of low-impact aerobic activity.**

What I'd like to do now is to break these down in more detail and show you the benefits of each system.

Then, we will look at how to apply them to our daily lives.

The 1st W – Weight Training

You begin to lose strength at 35 years old.

There are numerous benefits to a properly designed resistance weight training program. I like to explain these benefits in terms of primary and secondary. Here's why:

Many times people use tools for the wrong job.

The primary benefit of strength training is building strength and muscle.

This is how to use the weights properly.

As stated previously, the major decline with aging is the loss of strength and muscle.

The major way to "fight back" is through resistance exercise. That can be in the form of going to the gym and using machines, dumbbells, and barbells. You can also use body weight exercise or combine them all together.

As a personal note, I love lifting weights.

When I was very young, about 9 years old, my grandpa took me to K-Mart to buy a gift for me. He got me a set of weights—the cement kind. It was named "Ultra K-Tron"! That makes me smile just thinking about it.

The weights were red. I'll never forget that gift, as it set a course for my life!

I took those weights home, put them downstairs, and had my first gym. I put up a punching bag and would go down there and workout religiously, but I didn't have any idea what I was doing.

I bought a weight training book by Franco Columbu and followed the 6-day routine he put together. That was my first phase of learning what not to do! Six days per week at 9 years old was a bit much. I didn't make any real gains, but I was determined and persistent.

I bought every muscle magazine I could afford, and slowly—over many, many years — I began to deduce what worked and what didn't.

Let's dig into the good stuff!

Secondary Benefits of Weight Training:

"If you think lifting weights is dangerous, try being weak."
- Anonymous

We've learned that the primary benefit of weight training is to build strength and muscle. Now let's look at the secondary benefits.

Weight training **improves cardiovascular endurance.**

SelectHealth.org puts it this way: *One of the biggest benefits of weight lifting is lowering the probability of life-altering heart attacks and strokes. A recent study shared by the journal Medicine & Science in Sports & Exercise showed that weight training may reduce the risk of a heart attack or stroke. If you regularly lift weights, you reap these benefits—even if you aren't regularly participating in aerobic exercise such as hiking or running.*

Because strength training increases lean muscle mass, it gives your cardiovascular system places to send the blood being pumped. This results in less pressure on your arteries, which helps reduce the chances of heart-related problems. With consistent strength training, you're likely to stay heart-healthy for years to come. [15]

It helps your heart—weight training is good for your heart.

When I was in my early 50s, I went to my doctor for my annual physical. My resting heart rate is very low and I attribute that to years of lifting weights. It can vary between 38–42 beats per minute. The average is 60–100 bpm.

My doctor said we probably should get you an EKG, so I went and scheduled it.

When the day came for the EKG, I went through the normal paperwork and tests. The nurse kinda overreacted when she tested my resting heart rate and it was under 40. She panicked and said, "There's something wrong with you." Which, by the way, is exactly what you want to hear from your medical professional.

She then asked me if I was a runner. I said no, but I lift weights regularly. She said, "Well, that wouldn't be the reason for the low heart rate." I explained to her that weight training was actually BETTER for your heart than running. She disagreed with me, and I just simply let it go, knowing she was wrong!

She then called the doctor. He came in, and after she explained my "dilemma" to him, he simply said, "Well, let's get him hooked up and take a look."

Now, it's off to the treadmill with all kinds of wires hooked up. I started walking, nut they couldn't get my heart rate up enough for the test to work, so they put it on an incline. I' was now on an ascending incline, but I still couldn't get my heart rate up. "Start jogging," the wicked nurse instructed me. In my mind, I said, "You need to start jogging!"

But jogging it was. Still not the heart rate they wanted. "Start running," Nurse Annie Wilkes said. (Some of you will get the reference.)

So, I started running. I was running as hard as I could uphill, the treadmill timer was at 13 minutes, and my legs were on fire! But I wasn't going to let anyone know that, so I just powered through.

Finally, the doctor came back into the room and said, "Shut him down." He then told me that if something was wrong with my heart, it would've definitely shown up already. In his professional opinion, he said I was fine.

I wanted to look over at the nurse and do the 'I told you so' thing, but I didn't.

However, here's the best part of the story: she looked at me and asked me for a business card!

Weight training releases myokines.

ScienceDirect.com: *A single bout of exercise is likely to induce small to large increases in myokine expression immediately after and up to 60 min post-exercise, while myokine responses typically revert to baseline levels from 180 minutes to 24 hours post-exercise* ...[16]

I also read this:

Some myokines are thought to induce anti-inflammatory responses with each bout of exercise and mediate long-term exercise-induced improvements in cardiovascular risk factors, having an indirect anti-inflammatory effect.

The effects of resistance weight training and the release of myokines are far-reaching throughout the body. What this means is a properly performed resistance session will not only benefit your muscles, but also support your kidneys, heart, liver, etc.

This is why it's not only ok but also important to state...

Proper exercise is medicine!

Weight training **increases resting metabolic rate.**

Adding one pound of muscle can burn up to 30 extra calories per day. It'll depend on the individual to get an exact amount burned but we do know it helps the metabolism. I've read elsewhere that one pound of muscle gain will burn 6-10 extra calories per day.

Why the discrepancy? I have read of the metabolic benefits of muscle mass and while muscle doesn't dramatically increase your calorie output at rest, it does add significantly to your overall metabolic rate, especially when combined with other activities.

I have a client who is 60 and started training with me a few years back. One day, I saw him at church and thought, "Wow, he really looks different." I had seen him regularly in the gym and noticed his strength levels increasing, but he always wore loose-fitting clothes.

That day at church, he was dressed up, and his increased muscle mass was clearly noticeable. It made an incredible difference in how he looked.

When I mentioned it to him, he thanked me and told me he wasn't watching his diet closely but really noticed that his clothes fit so much better!

Simply working hard and gaining some muscle really made a difference for him.

Weight training **enhances mental health.**

Another way to put it is that weight training reduces depression and anxiety.

Exercise increases the endorphin response which helps our moods.

I have had several therapists refer clients with depression to me as they knew how much resistance training helped with moods.

Nearly every day, I'll have a client come in for a session and tell me how much they really needed to train. They find it removes the day-to-day stressors of life.

On a personal level, I find it necessary to train regularly and get outside to walk as well. As I'm typing this now, I've had a few days off from training because I've been out of town. The weather has also not been conducive to getting outside and taking walks. I'm noticing a couple of interesting things happening:

The first is stiffness. My legs are a bit stiff as I get up and down from the chair.

The second thing I notice is lack of focus, almost like a mental fog.

I'll go lift today and do my evening walk and I'm sure I'll feel better.

Another benefit in this category is how resistance training helps fight Alzheimer's and dementia.

A study conducted by the University of Sydney revealed the following: *The long-term study found that strength training led to overall benefits in cognitive performance, benefits linked to protection from degeneration in specific subregions of the hippocampus. The hippocampus is a complex structure in the brain with a major role in learning and memory.* [17]

Weight training is medicine for my brain!

Weight train also delays or reverses osteoporosis.

WebMD reports: *Did you know that weight training for osteoporosis—not just walking or doing aerobics, but lifting weights —can help protect your bones and prevent osteoporosis-related fractures? Studies show that strength training over a period of time can help prevent bone loss—and may even help build new bone.*

I have an exercise machine in my gym that measures the force when you push against it. You don't move in the machine once you get set up. You just push against the handles and as you do, the force you put out is measured and stored to compare against the next performance.

The theory behind the workout is based on creating greater forces on both the muscles and the bones thereby creating osteoblasts which build bone density.

A lot of people think osteoporosis is a women's-only problem, but it's not—it affects men as well. For that reason, I address it with both my male and female clients.

Dr. Doug McGuff talks about this in his book *Body By Science* and in a website [18] on inroad theory. *"Exposure to heavier weights causes microscopic cellular damage that initiates muscular adaptation and seems to be essential for stimulating increases in both muscle and bone mineral density."*

When he states "stimulating increases in both muscle and bone mineral density," he means that proper weight training builds your bones!

Last benefit of weight training: it **demotes diabetes.**

For people with diabetes, strength training helps the body respond better to insulin, improves the way it uses blood sugar, and lose weight.

Resistance training increases heart rate and respiration. During this process, muscles utilize more glucose that's circulating in the bloodstream, which can, over time, lower blood sugar levels.

Two randomized trials each found that resistance training, when coupled with calorie counting and weight loss, lowered the risk of progression from glucose resistance to Type 2 diabetes by approximately 58%. Researchers hence concluded that increased physical activity and modest weight loss decrease the likelihood of increased diabetic conditions.

My conclusion is that combining weight training and walking with a proper diet can really help reverse Type 2 diabetes.

My Take on Weight Training

At this stage of my life, I still love to lift weights!

I love to train and I love exercise and the way it makes me feel.

However, I've had to adjust so much of my own exercise. No longer do I train to "get bigger muscles."

I now train to "not lose muscle."

There's no difference in the training but there's a big difference in the mindset.

My mindset is everytime I go into the gym to train, I'm training with perfect form, total concentration, and I'm thinking safety first.

Another thought is my motivation. I read years ago lifting weights provides 56 benefits. I use that as a tool.

Here's a little self-talk for you that I use: "I'm going to take some medicine right now that has zero side effects and only positive benefits—56 of them."

The 2nd W – Walking

"If you seek creative ideas, go walking. Angels whisper to a man when he goes for a walk." – Raymond Inmom

Years ago I was walking at the St. Louis Mills Mall. This was when it was just being built. There were stores still available and they had canvas covering with writing on them.

As I walked, I saw the quote from Raymon Inmom from above. I just found it very interesting. I'm not saying it's theologically correct, but I am saying there's something to going for a good walk and clearing your mind.

Someone said, "Never to trust an idea that comes to you sitting down." That has been my experience. Whatever is on my mind becomes clearer while I'm walking.

This is where your physical health helps your mental health. It's another great way to fight the mental battle.

When I walk, I use it for my prayer time or for listening to sermons or worship music. There are times when I'll be on my treadmill and I'll watch educational videos.

The primary benefit of walking is to improve or maintain your health.

Walking also has secondary benefits.

Secondary Benefits of Walking

Here they are:

Walking improves heart health.

The National Heart Foundation of Australia estimates that walking 30 minutes or more each day can reduce the risk of stroke by a whopping 35 percent.

Walking lowers stress and improves mood.

Walking releases endorphins, a feel-good chemical in the body that promotes a state of pleasure like laughter and love.

Walking reduces depression.

Depression affects millions of people globally and is a leading cause of disability worldwide. Here's my insider tip with depression and walking. When you're walking, bring your phone and take pictures of beauty—anything that catches your eye.

I own a Jiu-Jitsu academy with my son, and we host people from all over the world for seminars. When they visit, they stay at my home.

There's two guys that come in on occasion, Chris and Charles, and they love the area. They do morning walks, and one morning Charles came back in and showed me the pictures of obscure flowers that he'd come across. I found that moment to be fascinating as I never looked for anything like that nor did I expect a tough Jiu-Jitsu black belt to be looking for them either.

Now when I go out for a walk, I observe and take pictures at times!

Walking helps your joints.

Researchers found that people who walked for exercise had a 40 percent reduction in knee pain when compared to a group that didn't walk.

Walking controls your blood sugar.

Those who walked regularly had a 30 percent lower risk of developing Type 2 diabetes.

Walking boosts immune function.

Walking may flush bacteria from the lungs and airways, reducing your chances of picking up cold and flu viruses. [19]

Walking also renews your sense of wonder.

When I talk about wonder, I'm talking about thinking differently.

We have so much information available through the internet, video, and media. Having that much information can cause us to lose our sense of wonder instead of inspiring us to explore it. I like to approach life with curiously.

One of my traits—and I don't know why I do this (I'm actually wondering why)—is that I tend to look at what everyone else is doing and then do the opposite. I think it comes from my life's experience of noticing that most people take the easy route rather than challenging themselves.

I didn't hear much about this growing up, but in our society now, we face a lot of issues with mental health. There are plenty of reasons for this, but much of it stems from the overload of information at our fingertips. We get alerts on our phones about the latest disaster in another country, access to social media showing us what everyone else is doing and how great their lives seem, while we're struggling to make ends meet. By the way, most people exaggerate how great their lives are. We're bombarded with an overload of news media, and it triggers us over and over again.

My suggestion: take a leisurely walk for 30 minutes per day— after dinner if possible. If that's not feasible, just walk whenever you have the time. This will aid in digestion and boost your metabolic rate. Some people like to count steps, which is fine. General guidelines suggest aiming for 4,000–10,000 steps per day.

My Take on Walking

I walk nearly every day. Sometimes I walk outside by myself, other times with Jen, or if the weather is bad, I'll use the treadmill.

Generally, I'll walk 30 minutes per day, but sometimes in the summer, I'll walk twice a day. I do it because I enjoy it. The 30-minute daily walk is part of my routine, and one super-secret trick is knowing when to walk.

he best time to walk is right after dinner. If you take a 30-minute walk within 15 minutes of finishing your dinner, you can increase your metabolic rate by 25–30%, according to Dr. Ellington Darden. [20]

When you walk after dinner, it also keeps you from going to the couch and craving more food.

After spending some time together, my cousin asked me how I felt both full and satisfied with the way I ate. I explained to him that those two things are mutually exclusive.

The full feeling comes from eating foods that are nutritionally dense and high in fiber. It also comes from the hormonal response triggered by walking after my meal.

As for being satisfied, it's different. I feel satisfied after my meals because I genuinely enjoy the foods I eat. That's not always the case for everyone. For some, satisfaction isn't about feeding the stomach—it's about feeding the brain. Here's what I mean:

Eating foods that are high in nutrition and fiber fills you up. However, those foods are not addictive, so they don't always satisfy you if you have food addictions.

When you eat certain foods—sugary foods, chips, or processed snacks—they release dopamine in your brain. That's how you become addicted to certain foods. Your stomach might actually be full (although some people don't know what that feels like), but your brain craves the rush of dopamine to feel satisfied.

Dr. Rob Cywes [21] talks about food addiction on YouTube and I've learned from his videos on how this addiction works.

I've seen this over and again, but on one occasion, I watched a small child put their hand in some sugar. They then licked the sugar and almost immediately their other hand tightened up and their body shivered. It was really interesting to watch. I was thinking this is when the addiction starts.

Walking will also aid in the digestion of your food.

When I walk right after my meal something very interesting happens. At about the seven minute mark, I'll notice some minor burps. At the 12 minute mark, I can feel my stomach begin to move things around. It's almost like clockwork.

After a while, I'll really have some big burps.

I can attest how much walking helps my digestion.

My suggestion is to make walking or some other form of low impact aerobic activity a part of your daily life.

What I mean by low impact aerobic activity is anything that doesn't hurt your joints. For example, riding a bike or using an elliptical. I'm not a fan of jogging, as it's very stressful on the joints over time.

One more walking thought:

Keep your pace leisurely. You don't have to walk fast to get the benefits. Sometimes walking too fast can actually cause some harm.

I had a client who was complaining of back pain and planning to visit a surgeon. I repeatedly asked her if she was doing anything that could have contributed to her pain, but she kept insisting she wasn't.

After a few sessions with me, I asked her to point out where the pain was, and she indicated her hip area.

I then asked if she was walking at all, and she said she was walking on a treadmill.

Bingo! That was the problem.

This is very important, so read slowly:

Do not allow the treadmill to dictate the speed of your walk. Make sure you walk at your normal pace and maintain that speed.

She had been walking way too fast, which disrupted her normal gait and caused inflammation.

Once she iced her hip and took some time off, the pain went away. When she resumed walking at a slower pace, the pain never returned.

Think about that. She might've had surgery, but it could have been a complete disaster for her.

We saved her a ton of trauma by examining what she was doing!

The 3rd W - Watching Your Diet

"More and more data reports that sugar is probably the most consumed addictive substance throughout the world and can be considered the new cocaine owing to its dramatic parallels and overlaps with drug-like effects. Both stimulate our brain's pleasure centers." - NextLevelUrgentCare.com

This is the biggest area of confusion, concern, and complaints for most people!

Confusion: People don't really know the basics of diet.

Concern: People are concerned about their health.

Complaints: People will come and tell me, "I don't eat that much."

All this is common, so we need to be educated. I want to begin by giving you some very important information.

I'm going to overview my eating ideas and then expound on them. I also want to look at a few things, such as:

- **Calories matter**
- **Fiber is very important**
- **Real food is best**
- **Intermittent Fasting works**
- **Hormones affect appetite**

But first, let's look at **the primary benefit of watching your diet.**

The primary benefit of watching your diet is that it helps reduce or control body fat levels.

Body fat levels aren't controlled by exercise, they're controlled by diet. That doesn't mean that exercise doesn't help. It's very important to use proper exercise along with your fat loss program.

Here's how it works.

Diet without strength training exercise equals weight loss. This weight loss includes body fat, muscle, and possibly bone.

Diet with strength training exercise equals fat loss. Most of the weight you lose, if you strength train, will be fat. Based on your level of strength training, you might lose a little muscle or in some cases even gain muscle.

Someone who never lifted weights before could start a program with a calorie-restricted diet and actually gain muscle and lose fat. It's not the norm, but it does happen.

Let me give you a wisdom tip:

You can't out-exercise a bad diet.

Dr. Ellington Darden, in his book, *Killing Fat*, writes,

"In spite of what some popular authors would have you believe, the laws of thermodynamics are constant. All things in nature—including human metabolism—are governed by thermodynamics. One gram of

carbohydrate and 1 gram of protein each contain 4 calories, while 1 gram of fat contains 9 calories. All calories from carbohydrates, proteins, and fats count toward the surplus, or deficit, of fat metabolism. Once it is consumed, there is no way to weaken, discount, or bypass a food's calories. To lose fat, you must consume fewer calories than you burn each day. Your calories per day should not be too low, or your body may pull nutrients from your muscles and vital organs, which is not desirable. The majority of people I've worked with achieve optimum fat-loss results by adhering to daily calorie levels that range from 1,800 to 1,400 for men, depending on body size, and 1,500 to 1,200 for women." [22]

The Secondary Benefits of Watching Your Diet

"With long life, I will satisfy him and show him my salvation."
- Psalm 91:16

Watching your diet can lengthen your lifespan.

Years ago, I read a book by Dr. Roy Walford. He was a physician and gerontologist known for his work on extending lifespan through dietary restriction. He was a pioneer in this movement that is still being studied today.

The name of the book is *The 120-Year Diet: How to Double Your Vital Years*, published in 1986. [23]

In this book, he discusses the concept of caloric restriction and its potential impact on aging and longevity. Dr. Walford believed that reducing calorie intake **without malnutrition** could extend human lifespan.

It is my opinion, he was and still is correct.

Here's why:

Eating less food reduces the stress placed on your organs. Add to that some intermittent fasting, and you have a prescription for health!

The only thing that slows aging is reasonable caloric-restriction with proper nutrition.

Watching your diet can augment awareness.

Watching your diet can keep you mentally focused.

Think about a time when you ate a heavy meal for lunch and about an hour later you just catch yourself yawning and almost groggy.

Barry Sears said, *"Food is one of the strongest drugs in our society."*

Watching your diet can elevate your emotions.

Eating right makes me feel better!

My Take On Diet

If you keep healthy food in your fridge, you'll eat healthy food.

Diets work! For a while.

Most people go back to the random eating that caused the weight gain after going on a "diet."

The reason is you can't live in deprivation for too long. Your hormonal responses will cause your body to go back to a certain weight setpoint. I've been through this personally for many years. It's called yo-yo dieting. Going up and going down with my weight. Restricting my foods for a period of time and then binge eating to put it back on.

This is why it's so important to develop a lifestyle of waiting that you can enjoy, lose the weight, and keep it off.

By the grace of God, that's what I've been able to do. My current eating lifestyle happened almost by accident—or perhaps by an answer to prayer.

Here's how it happened:

I was all in on the keto diet. It was working for me, but it was a bit of a struggle to stick with—still, I stayed on it.

One day I was eating something and when I bit down, a cap came off my tooth. I went to see my dentist and he tried to put it back on but said there just wasn't enough tooth left to do so. He suggested getting it extracted and putting in an implant.

I followed his advice and went to the oral surgeon.

As a side note, dentistry causes me A LOT of anxiety. I will break out in a sweat just going in.

I went to the oral surgeon and he started the extraction and it wasn't going well. I could hear my tooth cracking and breaking and then I look up at the monitor and noticed my blood pressure and pulse rate were dropping and everything was closing in on me.

My first thought was, "There's no way I'm going out by tooth extraction! I will not have my headstone read: 'He died getting his tooth pulled.'"

After a while, the tooth came out and it was about eight months or so before I got the implant.

During that time, my mouth felt so odd. It was like the Grand Canyon between my teeth. And everytime I ate meat, it would get caught in that canyon. It was super frustrating and because I'm so sensitive in that area, there was a lot of pain.

It was at that time I decided to just not eat meat for a while and go with easier foods on my mouth.

My diet consisted of a daily protein shake with fruit and almond milk, beans and rice, veggies, grains, and little to no meat.

I then started noticing something really strange: my taste buds were changing, and I loved the foods I was eating. Not only that, my joints felt better, my sugar cravings were gone, I was thinking more clearly, and my body fat levels were declining.

After the implant was in, I decided to stick with what I was doing since I had my annual doctor's visit coming up in two months, and I wanted to see how my blood work would look.

When I got my blood work back, my numbers were great, and my cholesterol was down. It wasn't necessarily high before, but it did go down.

The foods I eat now are ones I really enjoy, and I'm never stuffed or bloated—I just feel really good.

I've added meat back into my diet since my taste buds have returned a bit. I just don't eat too much of it—6 to 8 ounces at a time is plenty for me.

That doesn't mean there's no discipline involved in what I do because there is. You have to plan and have an idea of how to approach this.

There's a secret, and it's this: it's what you eat!

If you eat the right foods (foods that are filling yet lower in calories), you can live satisfied and still lose fat.

How Hormones Affect Your Appetite

Learn to listen to the leptin.

I'm not exactly sure where I read this but it really changed the way I look at food. I took this information to my doctor and we had a lengthy conversation on it. Dr. Gray is really cool and very smart. When I go for my annual visit, he will spend about an hour just talking about nutrition and exercise with me.

There are hormones in your body that impact your hunger.

The two that I want to focus on are the hormones **ghrelin** and **leptin.**

These two hormones control the energy balance within the human body.

Ghrelin is the hunger hormone.

Leptin is the full hormone.

Here's how I explain it to my clients: When your stomach is empty, it will release ghrelin to let your body know that it needs food. When your stomach is full, it will release leptin to let your brain know it's full.

That's just a simple explanation. It's a bit more complex but I like to keep it simple, as it can get confusing.

Here's what's interesting:

The hormone response is fast for ghrelin and slow for leptin.

Ghrelin is a faster-acting hunger hormone released when you have an empty stomach. It measures the highest right before you eat and dips within 60 minutes following a meal.

Leptin takes 45-60 minutes to let your body know it's full.

Leptin mediates the full feeling.

It works to suppress food intake, letting the body know enough food has been ingested, and to stop eating.

"In a perfectly working body, ghrelin tells us to eat so we don't die of starvation, and leptin tells us when to stop," says Dr. Michelle Sands, hormone, metabolism, and epigenetics expert and author of Hormone Harmony Over 35.

Unfortunately, hormones sometimes find that perfect balance elusive.

"Leptin is a bigger player than ghrelin when it comes to weight gain and energy balance," Dr. Sands says. "It's closely tied to your thyroid and brain. When leptin is working well, we have a better metabolic rate, mood regulation, memory, brain function, and mental sharpness. When it's not, it can play a role in obesity, mood swings, and brain fog." In addition, Dr. Sands says that "Some people are genetically predisposed to release more ghrelin, and they get hungry faster as a result." [24]

This personal hormone discovery taught me something.

I now eat more nutritionally dense foods instead of calorie-dense foods.

Calorie-dense foods contain a higher number of calories per serving.

Nutritionally dense foods contain more water, fiber, vitamins, minerals, and other important nutrients.

The goal for long-term fat loss is this: learn to eat more nutritionally dense foods than calorie-dense foods.

Here's an extreme example:

Compare the nutritional and calorie value of a Snickers bar to an apple. A small fun-size Snickers bar has about 100 calories, just like an apple. If I'm trying to fill my stomach with more nutrition and fewer calories, the apple is the go-to choice every time!

Which leads me to…

Calories matter.

Calories Matter

Don't Just Count Calories, make Every Calorie Count – Pinterest (Side Note – Please don't revoke my man card for quoting Pinterest)

Years ago, there was a guy who did what he called the Twinkie diet. [25] His name was Dr. Gary Haub.

He was a professor who set out to show that the food you eat doesn't matter as much for weight loss—it's more about the number of calories consumed.

He decided to eat Twinkies, Little Debbie snacks, and other sugary treats every three hours instead of traditional meals.

For some variety in his dessert regimen, he also added Doritos, sugary cereals, and Oreos. Despite eating mostly junk food (plus one protein shake per day), he limited his intake to 1,800 calories per day, about 800 calories less than what's needed to maintain the body weight of a man his size.

Interestingly, his body fat and cholesterol dropped on this diet, even though he was eating large amounts of fat and sugar. In other words, eating sugar and fat does not raise cholesterol, provided you are on a low-calorie diet and losing body fat.

We see similar findings in people who lose weight on the Atkins Diet. Their cholesterol levels improve even though they eat a diet very high in animal fat. This is because being overweight raises cholesterol.

Not surprisingly, Haub demonstrated what all doctors and scientists already know: weight loss is about the number of calories you consume, not the composition of those calories.

This is not something I recommend. I'm just making a point that calories really matter.

This is how I used to approach diet but once again it's not the best approach.

The truth is, it is more nutritionally sound to eat a fiber and nutrient rich, low-calorie, balanced diet than it is to eat a Twinkie diet.

However, the point I'm making is that calories really matter.

If you want to see more about this, I recommend that you take a look at a new study published in the *Journal of the American Medical Association.*

It'll show the same principles Dr. Haub used in his experiment.

To quote *The Wall Street Journal*: *The findings suggest that it matters little whether a diet is high or low in fat, carbohydrates or protein, it's calories that build body fat.*

Fiber

"The more fiber you eat, the leaner you're going to be."
- Clarence Bass, "Ripped 2"

Fiber helps "regulate the body's use of sugars, helping to keep hunger and blood sugar in check." Children and adults need at least 25 to 35 grams of fiber per day for good health, but most Americans get only about 15 grams a day. Great sources are whole grains, whole fruits and vegetables, legumes, and nuts.

Jeff Novick, Director of Nutrition at Pritikin Longevity Center wrote, "If there is any 'nutrient' that people are deficient in, it's fiber."

I try to eat a lot of fiber in the foods I choose and I also take a daily fiber supplement.

There are two types of fiber:

- **Soluble fiber.** Soluble fiber breaks down into a gel-like substance when you add water. It has many benefits including lower cholesterol and blood sugar levels. Soluble fiber is found in whole oats, psyllium husks, peas, beans and apples, as well as carrots and barley.
- **Insoluble fiber.** Insoluble fiber increases the bulk in your stool, which helps those who struggle with constipation or bowel irregularity. Vegetables lead the way here: cauliflower, green beans, and potatoes are good sources of insoluble fiber as well as wheat bran, nuts, and beans.

Here are the benefits of a high-fiber diet:

- **Regulates bowel movements.** This is very important as regular fiber intake reduces your chance of constipation.
- **Reduces bowel problems.** A diet rich in both forms of fiber can lower your risk of developing polyps, hemorrhoids, and

diverticulitis. Studies have also found that a high-fiber diet likely lowers the risk of colorectal cancer.

- **Realigns cholesterol levels.** There's both good and bad cholesterol and certain fiber found in oatmeal, most beans and bran may help lower total cholesterol levels by lowering LDL lipoprotein, or "bad," cholesterol levels. Studies also have shown that fiber rich foods may reduce inflammation.

- **Restores blood sugar levels.** Blood sugar levels can get out of control if you eat the wrong foods or if you have diabetes. Fiber—particularly soluble fiber—can slow the absorption of sugar and help improve blood sugar levels.

- **Recovers normal body weight.** Foods high in fiber or nutritionally dense foods seem to make us feel fuller than low-fiber foods, which can lead us to eating less and staying satisfied longer. Nutritionally dense foods means they have less calories for the same volume of food.

- **Redesigns the aging process.** Fibrous foods, especially cereal fiber—is associated with a reduced risk of premature death from cardiovascular disease and all cancers.

How much fiber do you need?

The Institute of Medicine, which provides science-based advice on matters of medicine and health, gives the following daily fiber recommendations for adults: Aim for 25-30 grams from food sources. [26] Supplements help but try to get most of your fiber from food!

One more thought:

Avoid extremes.

Don't try to go all in with fiber. It'll cause bloating, and can irritate your stomach. Start slowly and monitor your body's response.

Real Food Over Supplements

I take supplements daily, but the gist of my diet is real food!

The typical American diet is heavy in processed foods, refined grains, and added sugars, all of which come up short on essential vitamins and minerals. But even a healthy, well-balanced diet can fall short of needed nutrients, especially among older adults, reports the June 2015 *Harvard Health Letter.* [27]

"As we get older, our ability to absorb nutrients from food decreases. Also, our energy needs aren't the same, and we tend to eat less," explains Dr. Howard Sesso, an epidemiologist at Harvard-affiliated Brigham and Women's Hospital. [28]

It's best to improve the diet before using supplements, advises Dr. Sesso. That's because vitamins and minerals are most potent when they come from food. In food, they are accompanied by many other beneficial nutrients, including hundreds of carotenoids, flavonoids, minerals, and antioxidants that aren't in most supplements. Plus, food tastes better than supplements and is often less expensive.

An apple is a better choice than a protein bar. That doesn't mean you should never eat a protein bar—it just means real food should be your first choice!

I see weight loss programs where you have to buy the food from them and that's fine for convenience at times but it's no way to create a lifestyle.

Creating a lifestyle of eating means putting the effort forward to make sure you're prioritizing your health!

As far as what supplements to take, I would start with a simple daily vitamin and mineral supplement. You can branch out from there.

Water

Pure water is the world's first and foremost medicine.

There are a bunch of guidelines on water drinking. One that I've read about is the 8x8 rule on drinking water.

Drink eight 8-ounce glasses of water per day.

I've also read that most people are chronically dehydrated, which is probably true.

Here are some health benefits of drinking water based on evidence-based findings commonly cited, including from Healthline: [29]

- **Helps physical performance.** Staying hydrated is crucial for maintaining optimal physical performance, especially during intense exercise. Dehydration can lead to fatigue, altered body temperature control, and reduced motivation.

- **Maintain Energy Levels and Brain Function.** Even mild dehydration can impair various aspects of brain function, including mood, concentration, and memory. Drinking enough water helps maintain cognitive performance.

- **Prevents and Relieves Headaches.** Dehydration can cause headaches and migraines in some individuals. Drinking water can help prevent and relieve headache symptoms in many cases.

- **Aids in Digestion and Prevents Constipation.** Water helps break down food in the digestive system, ensuring smooth digestion and preventing constipation. Drinking enough water keeps your bowel movements regular.

- **Supports Healthy Skin.** Proper hydration helps maintain skin elasticity and prevent dryness. While it won't prevent wrinkles, it can keep your skin looking healthier and more radiant.

- **Helps Maintain Kidney Health.** Water helps the kidneys filter waste from the blood and excrete it through urine. Drinking enough water reduces the risk of developing kidney stones by diluting the salts and minerals in the urine that can cause stones.

- **Promotes Weight Loss.** Drinking water can boost metabolism slightly, helping to burn more calories. Drinking water before meals can also create a feeling of fullness, leading to fewer calories consumed.

One final tip: drinking ice-cold water can help you burn extra calories, according to UAMS Health.

Before You Begin

Caution: To warn

You are responsible for your health! Never forget this nugget of truth.

However, that doesn't mean there aren't people there to help you.

ALWAYS SEE YOUR PHYSICIAN BEFORE STARTING THIS OR ANY OTHER EXERCISE OR DIET PROGRAM.

Much care has been taken to confirm the accuracy of the information presented in this book; however, the author, editor, and publisher cannot accept responsibility for errors or omissions and make no warranty, express or implied, regarding its content.

The information in this book is intended for healthy men and women only. Individuals with health problems should not follow these suggestions without a physician's approval. Before beginning any dietary or exercise program, always consult your physician. Please follow the instructions outlined in this book carefully!

Once again, you—and you alone—are responsible for your health. I am here to guide you along the way, just as any medical professional would. Any fitness or medical professional can give you advice, but you make the final decisions about what you choose to do.

I encourage you to always verify any health advice, including mine, before acting on it. My goal is to equip you with enough information to understand the fundamental principles of sound health! With the help of your medical professional and this book, you can add quality years to your life.

Contraindications of Exercise

Systems of injury or overexertion

Contraindications to exercise are given so that you will be able to distinguish between the normal discomfort associated with exercise and any pain that could cause a legitimate concern.

The National Federal of Professional Trainers lists the following as contraindications to exercise: [30]

- **Joint Pain**
- **Excessive Sweating**
- **Dizziness**
- **Extreme muscle soreness**
- **Nausea**
- **Cramping**
- **Rapid Pulse**
- **Chest Pain**

If, during exercise, you experience any of the above symptoms, stop exercising immediately and consult your doctor.

PART 3 - THE PROGRAM
Understanding Principles

Principle #1 - Load

The principle of load dictates how you keep the targeted muscle under tension for the entirety of the set.

You can even say it's the principle of *loading the muscle*.

It's so important that we learn that one principle. It's a game changer and it takes practice.

Loading the muscle, or as some call it, continuous tension, is the cornerstone of my training philosophy and revolves around the idea of sustaining a constant load on the muscles throughout every repetition, creating a seamless flow of tension for optimal muscle engagement.

Understanding the significance of continuous tension is crucial for unlocking maximum muscle growth and strength. By consistently challenging your muscles throughout each set, you stimulate greater muscle fiber recruitment and foster more significant adaptations.

Here's how it works:

Let's take a bicep curl as an example.

When performing a bicep curl, focus on controlling the downward movement of the weight, resisting gravity at all times. Avoid fully extending your elbow, keeping a slight bend to sustain tension on the biceps and prevent relaxation between repetitions.

You simply keep the load on the muscle.

At all times throughout the exercise.

The exercise is finished when you can no longer move the weight in a SAFE fashion.

There's another tip to enhance the exercise even further:

It's the Mind-Muscle Connection:

With this method you can make the load feel even heavier and more effective by thinking about what's going on in the muscle during the exercise.

Feel what's happening. Be in the moment of the exercise. Focus on the sensations within their muscles and be mindful of maintaining tension throughout the entire set.

Cultivate a strong mind-muscle connection by consciously directing your attention to the targeted muscle group. Visualize the muscle at work, feel the contraction, and ensure a steady and deliberate pace to sustain tension and amplify the effectiveness of your workout.

The reason this works so well is you can actually take a moderately heavy weight and make it feel much heavier by simply focusing on the muscles. It takes practice but you get better at it.

Principle # 2 - Resistance

The principle of resistance dictates how much weight I should use on each exercise.

Using a weight that is excessively heavy can undermine the effectiveness of your workout.

Conversely, choosing a weight that is too light won't stimulate the muscle as deeply and thoroughly as needed.

Ideally, the optimal starting weight for an exercise is approximately 30 percent less than your maximum for 10 repetitions, in good form. For instance, if your maximum is 10 reps with 100

THE GOSPEL OF FITNESS

pounds, use 30 percent less, or 70 pounds for your workout. But there's a potential problem.

What if you don't know what your 10 rep max is?

If that's the case then simply start with a light weight and use good form. As you complete the higher number of reps, in good form, then simply add a little weight for the next workout. Just remember...

It's crucial to emphasize that your primary focus is on loading muscles, not on constantly lifting heavier weights.

Stick to your task—only increase the weight when absolutely necessary—and have confidence in the workout protocol to yield the desired results.

Here's the roadblock that you have to learn to get around:

You have to understand that strength is finite. It's not infinite, meaning there is a maximum level of strength you can reach by using weights in good form. That's one of the goals in our eight week program, to get you as strong as possible.

I'm no longer concerned about the amount of weight I lift as I get older. I'm more concerned about deeply stimulating the muscles I'm working. I still need a reasonably heavy load but not so much weight that I lose my feel for the movement.

We want to be under the load for a minimum of 8 reps and a maximum of 12 reps.

If I choose a weight that keeps me under the load for only less than 8 reps, that weight is too heavy. If I chose a weight that keeps me under the load for over 12 reps, then that weight is too light.

The sweet spot is 8-12 reps under the load.

What does that look like?

Let's take the pulldown as an example. I can do 8 plates in good form for about 12 reps at a rep speed of 3-4 seconds up and 3-4 seconds down.

When I slow down my rep speed and focus on loading my muscles, I recommend a lighter weight to begin with.

My reasoning is it helps me to load the muscle perfectly.

With that said, I'd use 6 plates on my pulldown when I start my workout. I also keep accurate records of my workouts and I do that by writing them down. I'll try to get back to that 12 rep goal but I do it slowly and...

I keep track of my weights and reps and record that in my journal.

If I can do 12 reps at slow speed and load the muscle perfectly then I'll add a small amount of weight on my next workout.

Note: There will be a point when you can't add any more weight and that's perfectly fine. It's actually what we want. When I get there, then I know I've done everything I can to keep loading that muscle better.

Principle #3 – Form

The principle of form dictates that controlled movements are the safest and most efficient way to stimulate muscle.

When I go out of town, I'll usually go to a gym for a workout. I'll generally mind my own business but it's very hard for me to do at times.

A few months back, I was in the gym and there was a guy doing a chest press. He probably did 20 reps in about 15 seconds. He was throwing the weight up and down without a purpose.

If you go to a gym, I want you to simply observe what's going on.

Almost every person you see training will be almost throwing the weights back and forth.

All the lifting and the lowering is too fast. Little, if any thought, is given to feeling the movement at all.

Here's what I want you to do:

I want you to go **SLOW** and **SMOOTH** with your movements.

I want you to raise the weight in 3-4 seconds and lower the weight in 3-4 seconds.

This is the principle of load that we talked about earlier. Just don't get bogged down by rep speed as it can take away from the focus of the exercise. Just move slow and controlled.

The idea is to keep the muscle under load or tension for the entirety of the set.

This will create a deep muscular burn.

As I tell my clients, "Just stay in it for as long as you can or until muscular failure," so stay in it!

What we're focusing on is:

Emphasizing the tension in the muscle.

You will really notice it. The idea is to really stay present in the moment for your workout but also to keep the muscle loaded as much as possible.

Another thought is do not slam, bounce, or jerk the weight in the critical turn-around transitions. The turn-arounds are when the movement shifts from lifting to lowering and then from lowering to lifting. Keep the turn-around transitions smooth and your results will be significantly improved.

Do not confuse demonstrating strength with building strength. Building strength is your goal. And building strength is most effectively produced by applying slow, smooth form in all your lifting and lowering.

Principle #4 - Intensity

The principle of intensity dictates how much muscular force you are momentarily capable of using.

Exercise intensity refers to the level of effort applied during a workout, focusing on reaching momentary muscular failure—the point at which you can no longer perform a repetition with proper form.

Intensity is measured by how close you push your muscles to failure within a controlled, slow-tempo repetition. The goal is to maximize muscle fiber recruitment and stimulate muscle growth in the most efficient way possible.

Intensity is a skill that is learned. You'll learn to push yourself during your workouts. Here's the idea: use perfect form for all your reps, and when you can't complete another rep with proper form, terminate the set.

This is the principle of intensity when lifting weights: train as close to muscle failure as possible while maintaining good form. If I were to sum up intensity, it's this: work hard!

Muscle failure occurs when you continue pushing or pulling the weight until no additional movement is possible. If you've selected the correct resistance, this failure should happen during standard exercises between the 6th and 12th repetition.

Don't stop an exercise just because you've reached a specific repetition number—always try for one more rep, even if it feels impossible. Strive to continually increase your intensity.

As a side note, the range of motion (ROM) for an exercise varies depending on the movement. For example, calf raises have a shorter range of motion than leg presses, so the duration of each rep will differ based on the ROM.

Principle # 5 - Progression

The principle of progression dictates that workout intensity must gradually increase as the body adapts, thereby providing a greater stimulus.

How do we use this progression principle in our exercise plan?

Let's define progress first and then we'll talk about the limits of progress.

Exercise progression is a systematic approach to gradually increasing the demands placed on the body during resistance training to stimulate continuous muscle growth and strength gains. In the context of my system, progression is crucial because it ensures that the muscles are continually challenged and adapting, preventing plateaus and maximizing results.

Here are the key principles of exercise progression:

Increase the load: The idea here is fulfilling the upper end of the rep range provided.. We're looking at getting to 8-12 reps in good form with most exercises. When you reach the 12 rep range, in good form, then you should add the smallest amount of weight possible.

Increase the reps: I have outlined most rep ranges as 8-12 for most exercises. When you start lifting, it's important to start with a lighter weight to ensure good form. Keep track of the number of reps you can do, in good form, and then try to add a rep or two when you workout again.

Adding weight or reps are the primary methods of progression in the system, gradually increasing the weight or resistance used in exercises. This increase must be small and incremental, ensuring that you're still able to perform the exercise with proper form and reach momentary muscular failure within a set number of repetitions.

There's one more way to increase the intensity:

Reduce the rest between sets. Reducing the amount of rest between exercises is another way to progress. Shorter rest periods keep the intensity high and force the body to adapt to a more challenging workload.

There's a limit on strength gains. Strength is finite, it's not infinite. The goal is to get as strong as we can in every exercise while using good form. Once we get to the upper limits of our strength levels we then want to keep that strength for as long as we can. That ensures our muscles are as big and strong as they can be.

In order to adjust our weights when needed, we should also monitor and record progress. Keeping detailed records of your workouts, including weights used, repetitions performed, and the progression in tempo or intensity. This allows you to measure your improvements and adjust the difficulty of the workouts based on objective data.

Here's a simple look at how to record an exercise

Chest Press (Seat Setting 6) 90/8 S

Here's what that means to me: On the chest press machine, I performed 8 perfect reps with 90 pounds. I marked it with a S to indicate to me to stay at that weight for the next workout.

Principle #6 - Negatives

"Negative training has shown to be more effective in increasing muscular size and strength than positive-style training."
- British Journal of Sports Medicine (2009)

The principle of negatives dictates intentionally controlling and focusing on the negative part of the movement.

Most people just think of the positive part of the movement. I want you to think on the positive and the negative.

Learn to really focus on the negative part of the movement. The easiest way to understand the negative part of the movement is to think in terms of lowering the weight. Most people concentrate more on lifting than lowering and I want you to think about both but really, really focus on the lowering part of the exercise.

Here are some reasons to focus on the negative part of the movement:

- You can recruit more muscle fibers.
- Add extra stress to the muscle motor unit, which means great muscle stimulation.
- Works great for rehabbing injuries.
- Allows you to train less frequently and still get great results.
- Helps stabilize joints.
- Promotes greater work in less time, making training more efficient and promotes faster results.

Dr. Marc Roig and His Research: Marc Roig, PhD, is a professor in the School of Physical & Occupational Therapy at McGill University in Montreal, Canada.

He and his group researched data on eccentric exercise and concluded that it was a more effective way to train your muscles.[31]

I want you to make sure you focus on both the positive and the negative parts of the movement as thinking through both parts of the movement will really help you connect your mind to the muscle and create much deeper fatigue when performing the exercise.

Principle #7 – Duration

The principle of duration dictates the length of your workout.

The Duration principle emphasizes short, intense workouts with limited rest between exercises. It suggests that increasing the duration of muscle tension during a workout (by extending the time under tension for each set—see principle #1: Load) can lead to greater muscle growth and fat loss, even with relatively short workouts.

Bodybuilder Mike Mentzer once said, "You can train hard, but you can't train long." Another way to put it: you can't sprint for miles.

Duration refers to the total number of exercises you perform per workout. I've included a different number of exercises in each phase of the program to keep your body guessing about what's coming next.

Generally, the goal is to be under load for about 60 seconds. You can go a little longer or shorter, but aim for 60 seconds as the sweet spot.

At the top end, 9 exercises would require approximately 12–13 minutes, and I suggest moving quickly between exercises to build anaerobic endurance. A typical workout takes about 15 minutes.

From week to week, the number of exercises changes while the intensity remains high. The purpose of this approach is to push the limits during our 8-week program and achieve the best possible results in the least amount of time.

Principle #8 - Frequency

The principle of frequency dictates how often you work out.

Weight training every day is not advised because your muscles require approximately 72 hours of recovery time between workouts. A two-times-per-week frequency schedule proves nearly ideal for most people. And it's certainly ideal to combine with a reduced-calorie diet.

My training philosophy is time efficient and effective as well as safe and the workouts deeply stimulate muscles which create a need for longer recovery times and infrequent workouts.

This is very important because I don't want to spend all day in the gym. I want to get in and get my work done and get out.

Some people go to the gym as it's their social life.

I have things to do and if I can get just as good of results with less time, why wouldn't I?

Surveys on why people don't exercise show they just don't have the time. That can be an excuse if you're training for an hour a day, five days per week. I talk to people all the time who try to train like this.

It can become a part time job!

I'm offering a way to get fit and healthy in a fraction of the time! My workouts are short but intense.

I just had a guy who trained five days per week for almost two hours per day. I took him through a properly conducted high intensity program and he only lasted for three exercises. On the fourth exercise, he looked at me and I honestly thought he was going to start crying. I'm not kidding.

He said, "I've never felt anything like this!" More is not better, harder and briefer is better.

What we did in the workout deeply stimulated the muscles and here's where it gets interesting. Those muscles have to not only recover from the workout but they have to rest enough to grow.

Which leads me to my next principle.

Principle #9 – Recovery

The principle of recovery dictates the amount of time needed to recover from the workout.

In my opinion, the principle of recovery is the least understood concept in exercise science. For this principle to apply, we need to track our progress during workouts. If we feel good and notice we're getting stronger, we know we're on the right track.

However, if we don't feel as strong, our joints ache, or we lose enthusiasm for workouts, it's a sign that we're not fully recovered for the next session.

When we start the program, we standardize the number of sessions per week to three. As we improve at increasing the load on the muscles and raising the intensity of our workouts, we also increase the demands on our bodies.

That extra demand requires more recovery time, which is when the program becomes more individualized. You'll actually learn to recognize when you're ready to train again.

The goal is to balance intense effort during training with sufficient recovery to avoid burnout and ensure long-term progress.

It gets trickier as you begin to notice that, at times, your body feels better training less, while at other times you may want to add a workout back in when reducing to two sessions per week. Learn to experiment with recovery, but always make sure you feel fully ready for your next workout. You'll find that your workouts improve significantly when you hit that recovery groove.

Your body isn't static; it's dynamic. It adapts and adjusts to what we throw at it, but if we throw too much, our body will let us know—through how we feel and how we progress.

Principle #10 - Range

The principle of range dictates the range of motion of the exercise I am performing.

If possible, we want to perform exercises through a full range of motion, as this increases muscle engagement and growth.

It's important to perform exercises within the natural range that the muscle is designed to function. For example, in a bicep curl, you would fully extend your arm at the bottom to stretch the bicep, then curl the weight up, fully contracting the muscle at the top. This full range of motion creates maximum tension and allows for optimal muscle growth.

There are exceptions to using a full range of motion. Sometimes, you may lose the load on a muscle if the movement extends too far. In these cases, you must learn to feel the muscle being engaged throughout the entire exercise to achieve optimal results.

117

Another exception applies to individuals with injuries or joint issues. In these situations, simply modify the range of motion while maintaining controlled movements.

The principle of range also reduces the need for excessive stretching. By moving the joints through their entire range of motion, you promote strength across the full range and reduce stiffness. This is especially important as people age and experience reduced flexibility.

In some cases, individuals may want to stretch more simply because it makes them feel better. Feel free to stretch after your workout. Stretch your muscles until you feel a light pull—you don't need to stretch intensely. This light stretching helps retrain your central nervous system to allow your muscles to lengthen without unnecessary resistance. When you perform weightlifting exercises through a full range of motion, your joints will become more supple, and added stretching will provide additional benefits.

You can also stretch in the morning. A short 5-minute stretching routine will benefit your day and help clear your mind.

One of the most common phrases I hear is, "I'm sore because I forgot to stretch." Quite frankly, this isn't true.

What matters is building strength throughout the full range of motion of the muscle. When you have this, your body will be as flexible as it needs to be. If you enjoy stretching, feel free to do so, but always stretch after your workout—not before—when your body is warmed up.

Here are some thoughts on routines:

The Ten Commandments of the Routines

1. **Familiarize yourself with the routine you are using.** If you are training at home make sure you have a working knowledge of the home routine, if using the gym routine learn that as well. The best way to learn is to read each exercise illustration and practice without much weight.

2. **Train with weights no more than three times per week.** Always taking at least one day off between weight training days. Weight training stimulates the muscles to grow; the actual growth takes place during recovery. I find 3 times per week is a great starting point but eventually you'll need to go to two times per week.

3. **Start with light to moderate weights.** When you reach the high number described in the "rep range" part of the illustrations, add the least amount of weight possible the next time you workout. Try not to add so much weight you perform less than the lower number in the rep range. Reps are not as important as loading the muscle but we will learn more on that as we progress.

4. **Follow the routines as they are listed.** There is a method in the way the routines are set up. The only time you should change the routines is due to injury or limitations. If that is the case, don't try to work through your injury!

5. **Control the weight throughout the entire movement.** Never move faster, always slower. Generally 3-4 seconds up and 3-4 seconds down is best. If I shouted "STOP" in the middle of your exercise, the movement should halt easily. Using momentum to lift weights can cause injury. The actual time of the rep will be determined by the length of the exercise. A wrist curl has a shorter range of motion than a squat and will thereby have a short time during the rep.

6. **Perform only ONE SET of each exercise!** Doing more than one set is like driving down the same road twice. Train hard, and then get out of the gym!

7. **Don't waste time with excessive warm ups unless you feel you need them.** Too much warm up isn't necessary and can tire you out.

8. **Record your workout in your journal!** You need to keep track of your progress.

9. **Try to do better in either amount of weight lifted or number of reps performed.** But don't sacrifice proper form! Move from exercise to exercise as quickly as you can. I want your breathing to be elevated. Just try to develop a "flow" in your form. There will be a point where you can't do more weight or more reps and that's perfectly fine. Strength is finite, not infinite. I want to get you to the upper levels of strength safely. Once again...

10. **There will be a point where you can't lift any heavier weight.** When you hit that I want you to really focus on

the muscle. You'll learn to contract the muscle better with time.

There you have it: the Ten Commandments of the routines. What follows is an overview of the routines, then the exercise illustrations.

The Warm-Up

You can warm up before starting your workout, if you choose. Some people like to use an exercise bike for two minutes and then begin the program. Personally, I just get right into it, but I do visualize my workout beforehand by mentally rehearsing what I'm going to do.

The first exercise is abdominal work, which usually raises your core body temperature and gets blood flowing throughout your body.

As you begin handling heavier weights and learning how your body responds, your warm-ups will naturally adapt to suit you as an individual. Warm-up needs vary based on age, physical condition, weather, and the temperature of your workout space.

Be careful not to warm up so much that you exhaust the strength needed for your workout. As for the type of warm-up you choose, that's entirely up to you. You can use an exercise bike or any low-impact aerobic exercise, such as walking outside or on a treadmill.

The Cool-Down

You can also choose to include a short cool-down at the end of your workout.

Some people prefer to do their aerobic work after the workout, but that's a personal choice based on how much time you have. When I'm in serious weight-loss mode, I've found that I lose a bit more body fat if I do my aerobic work at the end of my workout—but I make sure not to overdo it.

I believe this is because body fat is burned when muscle glycogen levels are depleted. Resistance weight training depletes glycogen levels, reducing or even eliminating the time usually needed to deplete them with aerobics. As a result, you start burning body fat for energy immediately when you do aerobic work after weight training.

This is my own personal theory, and I haven't heard anyone else affirm it. However, it has worked well for me and others who have tried it.

Home Workout Plan

All exercises are one set of 8-12 reps, unless indicated (See Principle #5 - Progression).

Here's the workout plan: move from exercise to exercise with as little rest as possible.

The eight-week plan will look like this: during weeks one through three, we'll perform nine different exercises on three non-consecutive days of the week. We'll take at least one day off—sometimes two—between workouts to allow your muscles to recover. In this phase, we'll train three days per week to focus on learning proper exercise form.

After the initial three weeks, we'll make a few changes for weeks four through six. We'll add one exercise and drop one workout per week to account for the increase in strength you'll begin to experience. At this point, you'll be performing ten exercises per session, and you should start feeling stronger.

Most people think that getting stronger means they should work out more, but this is inherently incorrect. The stronger you become, the more demands are placed on your system, and you'll need more recovery time between workouts. As a result, we'll reduce the frequency slightly.

In the final two weeks, we'll stick to two workouts per week and add one more exercise to increase the overall demand on your body as we approach the final stretch.

Here's an outline of the plan, followed by the workout descriptions.

Weeks 1-3 - Workout 3 non-consecutive days (Ex. Mon-Wed-Fri)

- Plank (Hold for up to 60 seconds)
- Glute Bridge
- Db Squats
- Superman Row with a Towel
- Dumbbell Bench Press
- Dumbbell Side Lateral Raise
- Overhead Tricep Extension (Two-Hands on one Dumbbell)
- Dumbbell Bicep Curl
- Push-Up

Weeks 4-6 - Workout 2 non-consecutive days per week (Ex. Mon-Fri)

- Crunch
- Glute Bridge
- Db Squats
- Superman Row with a Towel
- Two-Arm Dumbbell Row
- Dumbbell Bench Press
- Dumbbell Side Lateral Raise
- Overhead Tricep Extension (Two-Hands on one Dumbbell)
- Dumbbell Bicep Curl
- Push-Up

Weeks 7-8 - Workout 2 non-consecutive days per week (Ex. Mon-Fri)

- Crunch
- Plank (Hold for up to 60 seconds)
- Goblet Squats
- Dumbbell Deadlift
- Superman Row with a Towel
- One-Arm Dumbbell Row
- Dumbbell Bench Press
- Dumbbell Side Lateral Raise
- Overhead Tricep Extension (Two-Hands on one Dumbbell)
- Dumbbell Bicep Curl
- Push-Up

Home Workout Exercise Descriptions

Exercise: Crunches

Target Muscles:

- Primary: Rectus Abdominis (the "six-pack" muscles)
- Secondary: Obliques, Hip Flexors

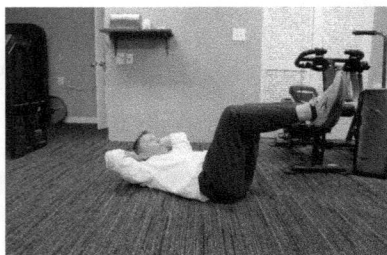

Starting Position

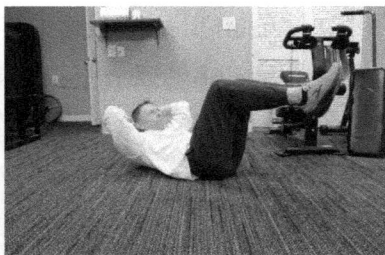

Ending Position

HOW TO DO THE EXERCISE:

1. Lie down on your back with your knees bent at 90 degrees with your feet in the air or planted firmly on the floor. Interlock your fingers and place them behind your head. Keep your elbows back and do not pull on your head. (See Starting Position)

2. Concentrate on flexing or contracting your abdominal muscles and slowly raising your shoulders and upper back off the ground. Pause in the contracted position and return to the starting position. (See Ending Position)

Exercise Tip: *When returning to the starting position, do not allow your head to touch the ground. In order to do this, you must keep your abdominal muscles contracted. This allows complete control of your upper body. Only let your shoulders lightly touch the ground. Also try to keep your lower back pressed into the floor as this maintains tension on your abdominal muscles.*

More Tips and Modifications:

- Easier: To reduce the intensity, perform the crunches with your feet resting on the floor.
- Harder: To increase intensity, hold a weight plate or dumbbell against your chest as you crunch.

Exercise: Plank

Target Muscles:

- Primary: Core (Rectus Abdominis, Transverse Abdominis)
- Secondary: Shoulders, Back, Glutes

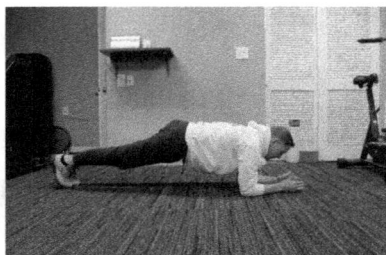

Starting/Ending Position

HOW TO DO THE EXERCISE:

1.Lie face down on a mat with your forearms on the ground. Bring your body off the ground with your toes tucked under and your feet shoulder width apart.

(See Starting Position)

2. There is no movement in this exercise so the starting and ending positions are the same. This is a static hold position.

Exercise Tip: *Really focus on what your abs are doing. You should feel some tension in the abdominal area. Adjust hand/elbow position to increase tension on your abdominal muscles.*

More Tips and Modifications:

- Keep your body flat to maximize the effectiveness of the exercise.
- Be aware of arching your back or letting your hips drop, which can reduce the effectiveness of the exercise.
- To make the exercise easier: Drop to your knees instead of your toes, or place your hands on an elevated surface like a bench or step.
- To make the exercise harder: To increase difficulty, try moving your elbows a few inches forward. This will increase the difficulty of the exercise.

Exercise: Superman Row with a Towel

Target Muscles: Lower back, upper back, shoulders, glutes, and hamstrings

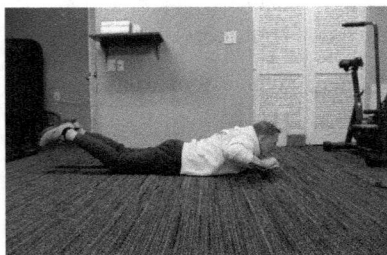

Starting Position   **Ending Position**

HOW TO DO THE EXERCISE:

1. Lie face down on an exercise mat, extend your arms in front of you, and keep the legs straight.

2. Hold a towel in your hands, keeping your arms a little wider than shoulder-width.

3. Lift your arms and legs by contracting your lower back muscles. (See Starting Position)

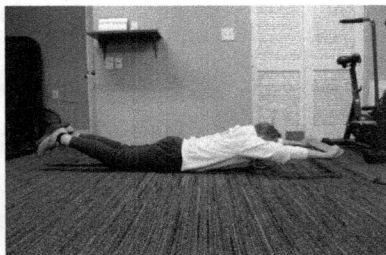

4. While maintaining the position, slowly pull the towel towards your chest by bending your elbows and squeezing your shoulder blades together. Think of the weight being on the backs of your arms as you slowly pull the elbows toward your waist.

5. Squeeze the muscles of your upper back together and hold this position briefly. (See Ending Position)

Exercise Tip: *Pause briefly and really try to squeeze the upper back muscles in the contracted position. When returning to the starting position, keep your head in the neutral position. There are several muscles contracting when you do this exercise which means you'll feel the muscle in more than one area.*

More Tips and Modifications:

- Avoid straining your neck by keeping your eyes slightly downwards.

Exercise: Dumbbell Bench Press

Target Muscles: Chest (pectorals), shoulders (deltoids), triceps

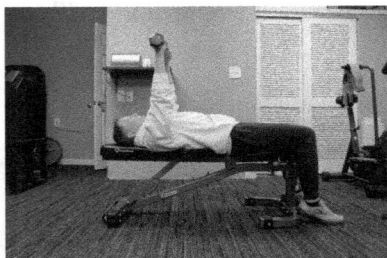

Starting Position

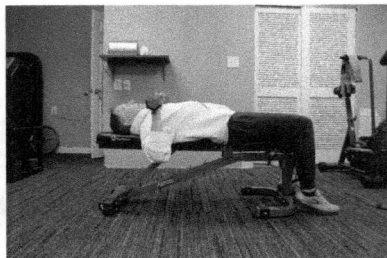

Ending Position

Getting into the position:

1. Sit on a flat bench, holding the dumbbells, one in each hand while they rest on your thighs.

2. Slowly lie back on the bench, bringing the dumbbells to your chest.

HOW TO DO THE EXERCISE:

1. Start with the weights above your chest, arms fully extended. (See Starting Position)

2. Slowly lower the dumbbells to your chest until you reach about an inch above the shoulders. (See Ending Position) Slowly push the dumbbells up and slightly inward, be careful not to let the dumbbells touch each other at the top of the movements. (See Starting position)

3. Return the dumbbells to your shoulders and start again.

Exercise Tip: *The dumbbells may feel shaky when you first start doing this exercise. Just make sure to move slowly and maintain control of the weights. Start with lighter weights and work your way up slowly. This will ensure safety.*

More Tips and Modifications:

- Make sure your shoulders remain in contact with the bench to avoid undue strain in your shoulders.

- Avoid flaring your elbows out too wide, as this can cause strains in the shoulders.

- If you don't have a bench you can use the floor. You'll reduce some of the range of motion of the exercise but you'll still get the benefit.

Exercise: Two-Arm Dumbbell Row

Target Muscles: Upper back (latissimus dorsi, rhomboids, trapezius), shoulders (rear deltoids), biceps, and core

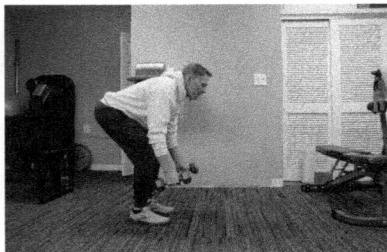

Starting Position   **Ending Position**

HOW TO DO THE EXERCISE:

1. Your feet should be shoulder-width apart, with a dumbbell in each hand. Your palms should be facing your body and your elbows should be close to your side. (See Starting Position)

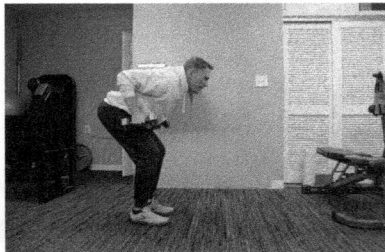

2. Bring the weight up and back. The dumbbells should travel in a line along your leg, not in a straight up and down line. Do not bring your elbow much higher than your hips, as this takes the stress off the lats, which is the target muscle. (See Ending Position)

Exercise Tip: *It's important in movements for your back muscles that you concentrate on getting the proper "feel" from your back and not your arms. In order to do this, imagine the weight pushing against the back of your arm or your elbow. Then think of hitting someone* *behind you with your elbow. When you get to the top of the movement, squeeze the shoulder blades together.*

More Tips and Modifications:

- Keep your back flat and your core engaged throughout the exercise to avoid placing strain on your lower back.

Exercise: One-Arm Dumbbell Row

Target Muscles: Upper back (latissimus dorsi, rhomboids, trapezius), shoulders, biceps

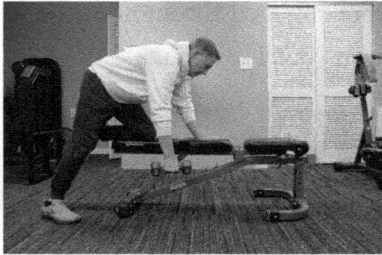

Starting Position   **Ending Position**

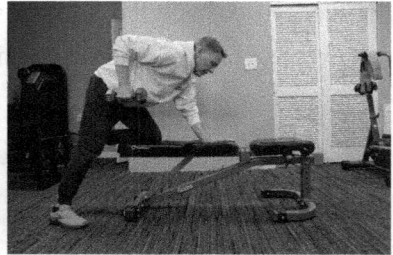

HOW TO DO THE EXERCISE:

1. Support your body by placing your right hand and right knee on a bench. Hold the dumbbell in your left arm with your arm extended toward the floor. Keep your elbow close to your side. (See Exercise Tip)

2. Bring the weight up and back. The dumbbell should travel in a line along your left leg, not in a straight up and down line. Do not bring your elbow much higher than your hips, as this takes the stress off the lats, which is the target muscle. (See Ending Position)

Exercise Tip: *It's important in movements for your back muscles that you concentrate on getting the proper "feel" from your back and not your arms. In order to do this, imagine the weight pushing against the* *back of your arm or your elbow. Then think of hitting someone behind you with your elbow.*

Tips:

- Avoid rotating your torso as you row the dumbbell; keep your shoulders level and stable.
- Use a weight that challenges your muscles but allows you to perform the exercise with proper form throughout all repetitions.
- Focus on the mind-muscle connection, particularly on contracting your back muscles as you lift the weight.

Exercise: Dumbbell Side Lateral Raise

Target Muscles: Shoulders (primarily the lateral deltoids)

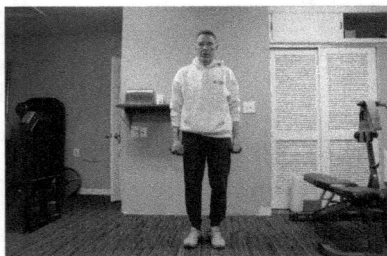

Starting Position   **Ending Position**

HOW TO DO THE EXERCISE:

1. Stand erect with a dumbbell in each hand, palms facing in. Keep your elbows slightly bent. (See Starting Position)

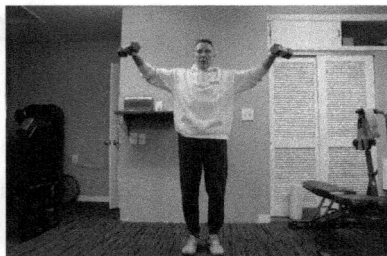

2. Begin to lift the weights out to the sides while leading with your hands and making sure you "feel" the shoulders work. Pause briefly at the top before returning to the starting position. (See Ending Position)

Exercise Tip: *Make sure that you don't rest too much at the bottom of the exercise. The movement is not directly out to the side but slightly in front of you. The slight pause at the top will increase the strain on the target muscles which is the shoulders.*

More Tips and Modifications:

- Keep your shoulders down and relaxed to avoid engaging your traps excessively during the lift.

- Start with a lighter weight to ensure you can maintain correct form, particularly if you're new to the exercise. Do not increase the weight load too much as you're working a small muscle group.

Exercise: Dumbbell Bicep Curl

Target Muscles: Biceps (biceps brachii)

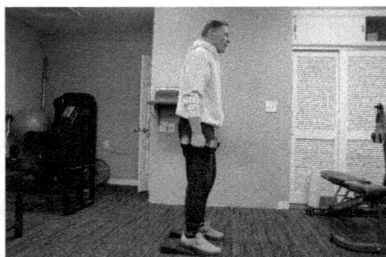

| **Starting Position** | **Ending Position** |

HOW TO DO THE EXERCISE:

1. Stand erect with a dumbbell in each hand, palms facing in. Keep your knees slightly bent. (See Starting Position)

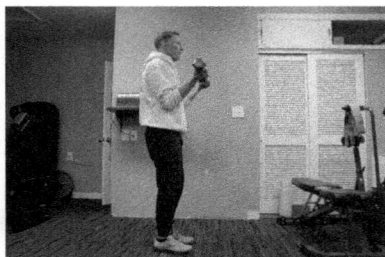

2. Begin to curl the weights upward at the same time, rotate your hands so that your palms are facing up. This happens at the midpoint of the movement. (See Ending Position)

3. Flex the biceps hand at the top of the movement. (See Ending Position) Return the weights to the starting position by rotating the dumbbells back to the starting position.

Exercise Tip: *Make sure that you don't let your elbows drift out to the side when you are lifting the dumbbells. This will increase the strain on your elbows and wrists and take the stress off of the target muscles (the biceps).*

More Tips and Modifications:

- Avoid swinging your body or using momentum to lift the weights; keep the movement slow and controlled to maximize bicep engagement.
- If you find yourself using your shoulders or back to lift the dumbbells, reduce the weight to maintain proper form.
- For added intensity, try pausing for a second at the top of the movement to fully contract the biceps.

Exercise: Overhead Tricep Extension (Two-Hands on One Dumbbell)

Target Muscles: Triceps (triceps brachii)

Equipment: One dumbbell

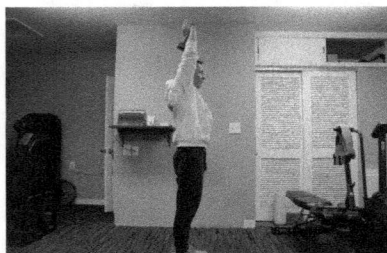
Starting Position

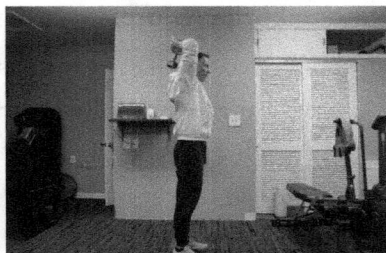
Ending Position

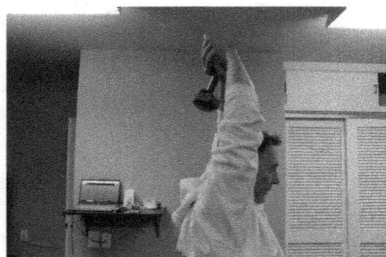
Grip Position

HOW TO DO THE EXERCISE:

1. Lift the dumbbell over the back of your head and place your palms flat against the dumbbell with one hand slightly overlapping the other. (See starting position)

2. Lower the dumbbell behind your head until you feel a good stretch in the back of your arms. Note: Let your elbows find their

own natural position for this movement. If you try to force them into a particular position, you put undue stress on the joint. (See Ending Position)

3. Return the dumbbell up to the starting position.

Exercise Tip: *Be very careful not to hit yourself in the back of the head with the dumbbell. In order to avoid this error, keep your elbows as straight up in the air (elbows toward the ceiling) as you can.*

More Tips and Modifications:

• Elbow Position: Keep your elbows pointing straight up and close to your head throughout the exercise to properly isolate the triceps.

Exercise: Glute Bridge

Target Muscles:

Primary: Glutes (Gluteus Maximus)

Secondary: Hamstrings, Lower Back, Core

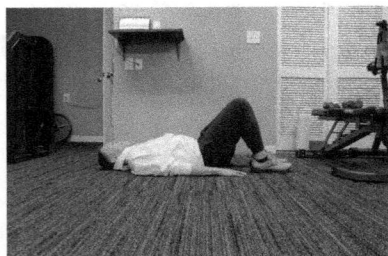

Starting Position   **Ending Position**

HOW TO DO THE EXERCISE:

1. Lie flat on your back on a mat or soft surface. Bend your knees and place your feet flat on the floor, hip-width apart, with your heels close to your glutes. Keep your arms at your sides, palms facing down. (See Starting Position)

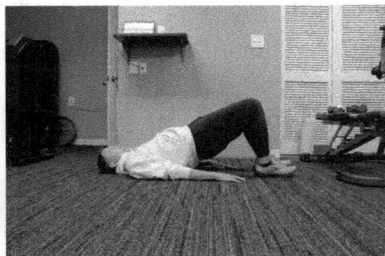

2. Press through your heels and lift your hips off the ground, creating a straight line from your shoulders to your knees. Squeeze your glutes at the top of the movement and hold for a moment, ensuring your body remains in alignment. Slowly lower your hips back to the starting position, controlling the movement to maximize engagement of your glutes and hamstrings.

(See Ending Position)

Exercise Tip: *Avoid arching your back excessively; focus on lifting with your glutes and not your lower back.*

More Tips and Modifications:

- To make the exercise easier: To reduce the intensity, place a pillow or rolled-up towel under your lower back for support or perform the bridge with your feet on an elevated surface like a step.

- To make the exercise harder: To increase difficulty, move your feet 2-3 inches further away from your waist and hold each rep for 5 seconds at the top of the movement. Squeeze the glutes during the hold.

Exercise: Goblet Squat

Target Muscles:

Primary: Quadriceps, Glutes

Secondary: Hamstrings, Core, Calves

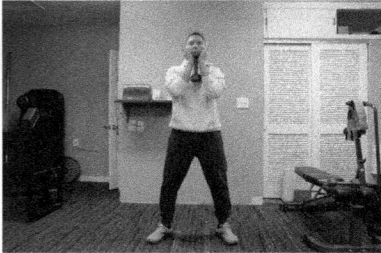

Starting Position   **Ending Position**

HOW TO DO THE EXERCISE:

1. Stand erect with one dumbbell in your hands with palms facing upwards and your feet slightly wider than shoulder-width apart. (See Starting Position)

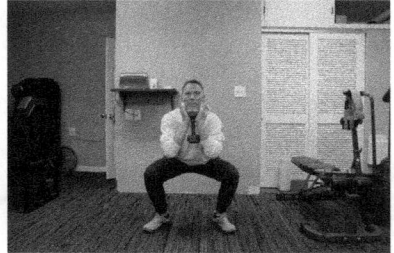

2. While keeping the heels on the floor, bend the knees and sit slightly back as if you were going to sit in a chair. When your thighs are parallel to the floor, (See Ending Position) begin to come back up slowly to the erect position, but not all the way, as you want to keep the muscle loaded.

Exercise Tip: *Always keep your back in neutral spine position (slightly arched) and concentrate on using your legs for the movement.*

If you think about pushing with your heels, as opposed to the balls of your feet, you will involve more of your lower body.

More Tips and Modifications:

- Keep your weight distributed slightly to your heels, to maintain balance and stability.
- Avoid letting your knees extend past your toes or collapsing inward.
- Maintain a neutral spine throughout the movement, avoiding rounding your back.

Exercise: Dumbbell Deadlift

Target Muscles: Hamstrings, glutes, lower back, core, and upper back

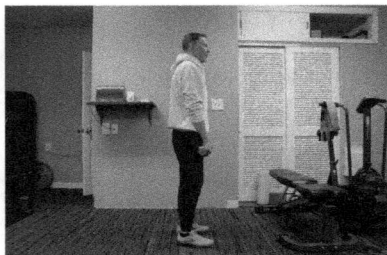

Starting Position   **Ending Position**

CAUTION: *If you have any lower back problems at all or if this exercise aggravates your back, please eliminate this exercise from your routine!*

HOW TO DO THE EXERCISE:

1. Stand erect with dumbbells in your hands, palms facing your sides. (See Starting Position)

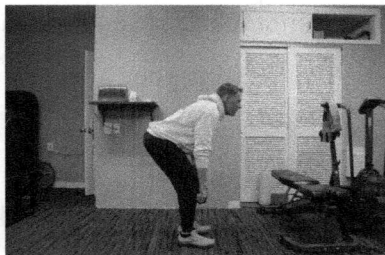

2. While keeping your back slightly arched, bend forward at the waist. Keep the dumbbells toward the front of your legs and only go down far enough to feel the stretch in your hamstrings. (See Ending Position)

3. Return slowly to the erect position but not all the way as you want to keep the muscle loaded.

Exercise Tip: *You should feel a good stretch in your hamstrings if you are doing the movement correctly. If you do not feel a good stretch in the hamstrings, try pushing your glutes and hips (butt) back a little more.*

More Tips and Modifications::

- Avoid rounding your back at any point during the exercise; maintaining a flat back is crucial for protecting your spine.
- Use a weight that allows you to maintain proper form throughout the entire range of motion without compromising your posture.

Exercise: Dumbbell Squat

Target Muscles: Quadriceps, hamstrings, glutes

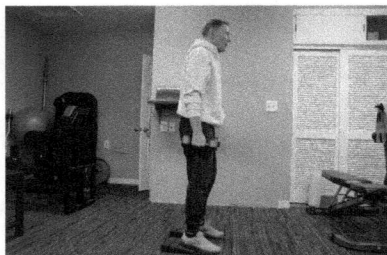

Starting Position   **Ending Position**

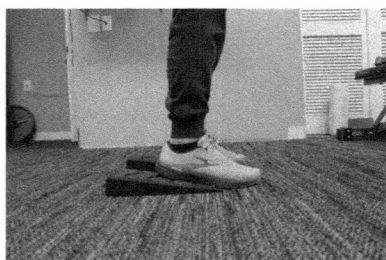

Inset

HOW TO DO THE EXERCISE:

1. Stand erect with dumbbells in hands palms facing in, feet shoulder width apart. (See Starting Position)

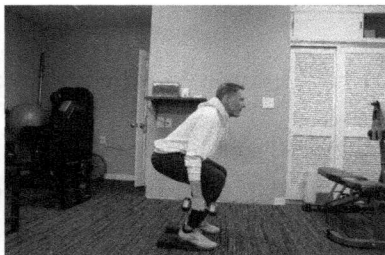

2. I use a heel lift as it helps keep the stress on my quads and off my knees. (See Inset)

3. While keeping the heels on the floor, bend the knees and sit slightly back as if you were going to sit in a chair. When your thighs are parallel to the floor, (See Ending Position) begin to

come back up slowly to the erect position but not all the way as you want to keep the muscle loaded.

Exercise Tip: *Always keep your back in neutral spine position (slightly arched), and concentrate on using your legs for the movement. If you think about pushing with your heels, as opposed to the balls of your feet, you will involve more of your lower body.*

More Tips and Modifications:

- Keep your knees aligned with your toes throughout the movement to avoid placing unnecessary strain on your knees.
- Keep your knees tracking in line with your toes as they will have a tendency to cave inward if you let them drift.

Exercise: Push-Up

Target Muscles: Chest (pectorals), shoulders (deltoids), triceps, core, and lower back

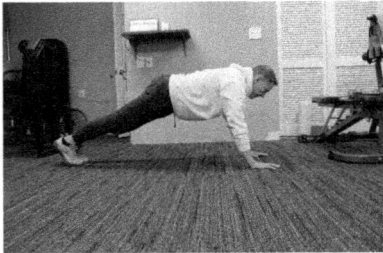

Starting Position

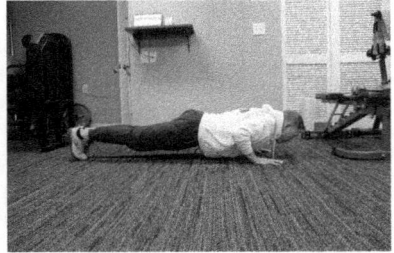

Ending Position

HOW TO DO THE EXERCISE:

1. Start with your arms straight, hands about shoulder-width apart, feet hip-width apart, palms and toes on the floor, and your body as straight as possible. (See Starting Position)

2. Lower your body slowly until you are almost touching the floor. (See Ending Position)

3. Push yourself up slowly to the starting position but stop before complete lockout.

Exercise Tip: *If the exercise is too difficult with the form described above, put your knees on the floor to make the workout more manageable. Then try to keep your hips/butt back near but not too close to your feet. This reduces tension on the upper body. As you get stronger you can move your hips forward which increases the intensity of the exercise.*

More Tips and Modifications:

- Elbow Position: Keep your elbows at a 45-degree angle from your body to protect your shoulders and maximize chest engagement.

Gym Workout Plan

All exercises are one set of 8-12 reps, unless indicated (See Principle #5 - Progression).

Here's the gym workout plan. Just like the home workout plan, move from exercise to exercise with as little rest as possible.

The gym workout eight-week plan will follow a similar structure to the home plan in terms of programming.

During weeks one through three, we'll perform nine different exercises on three non-consecutive days of the week. We'll take at least one day off—sometimes two—between workouts to allow your muscles to recover.

In weeks four through six, we'll add two exercises. This differs slightly from the home workout because we have more options available in the gym. We'll use those additional options to create more intensity in the plan.

In the final two weeks, we'll stick to two workouts per week and add two more bodyweight exercises to increase the overall demand on your body as we approach the final stretch.

Here's an outline of the plan, followed by the workout descriptions:

Weeks 1-3 - Workout 3 non-consecutive days (Ex. Mon-Wed-Fri)

- Machine Ab Crunch
- Calf Raise
- Leg Curl
- Leg Press
- Lat Pulldown
- Chest press
- Seated Row
- Overhead Press
- Machine Bicep Curl

Weeks 4-6 - Workout 2 non-consecutive days per week (Ex. Mon-Fri)

- Machine Ab Crunch
- Calf Raise
- Leg Curl
- Leg Press
- Leg Extension
- Lat Pulldown
- Chest press
- Seated Row
- Overhead Press
- Machine Bicep Curl
- Tricep Pressdown

Weeks 7-8 - Workout 2 non-consecutive days per week (Ex. Mon-Fri)

- Machine Ab Crunch
- Calf Raise
- Leg Curl
- Leg Press
- Leg Extension
- Lat Pulldown
- Chest press
- Seated Row
- Overhead Press
- Machine Bicep Curl
- Tricep Pressdown
- Inverted Rows
- Push-Up

Gym Machine Exercise Descriptions

Exercise: Machine Ab Crunch

Target Muscles: Rectus abdominis (the "six-pack" muscles), obliques

Equipment: Ab crunch machine

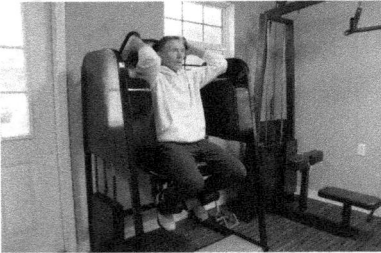

Starting Position   **Ending Position**

HOW TO DO THE EXERCISE:

1. Place both feet under the bottom pads of the machine. Grasp the handles with both hands. If the seat height is correct, your hands will be a little higher than your eyes. (See Starting Position)

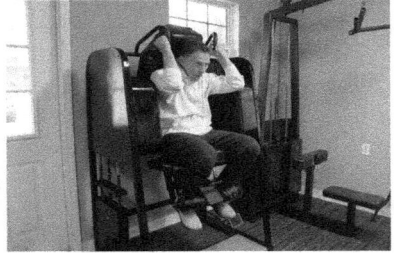

2. Slowly contract your abdominal muscles and curl your spine. Bringing your upper body closer to your lower body. (See Ending Position)

3. Lower the weight slowly but do not allow the moving weights to come in contact with the unused weight stack.

Exercise Tip: *The function of your abdominal muscles is to flex your spine. If you concentrate on your abs contracting while doing the exercise (i.e. feel your stomach tighten), you will get much better results.*

More Tips and Modifications:

- Start with a moderate weight. I've found that going too heavy causes bracing from other muscle groups. Lighter weights help you to perform the exercise with proper control.

- Make sure the movement is controlled, avoiding any fast motions.

- Keep your focus on the abdominal muscles throughout the exercise; this will help avoid pulling with your arms or using your legs to initiate the movement.

Exercise: Calf Raise

Target Muscles: Calves (gastrocnemius, soleus)

Equipment: Calf Machine

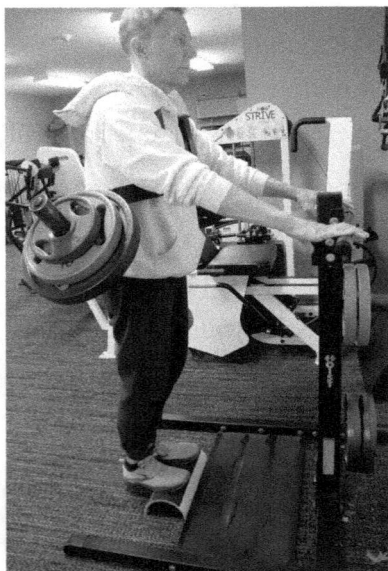

| **Starting Position** | **Ending Position** |

NOTE: Although machines for standing calf raises vary, the yoke of the machine will rest on your shoulders.

HOW TO DO THE EXERCISE:

1. With your knees slightly bent, adjust your shoulders under the pads of the machine. The balls of your feet should be on the edge of the step and in a stretched (lowered) position. (See Starting Position)

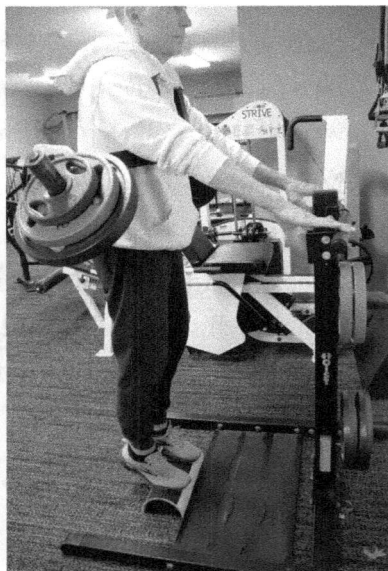

2. Push up off the balls of your feet until your heels are as high as they can go. (See Ending Position)

3. Return to the starting position.

Exercise Tip: *When you get to the top of the movement, try to go just a little higher. This will give you a good muscle contraction and make the movement just a little more effective!*

More Tips and Modifications:

- Use moderate weights to make sure you get the proper feel of the movement.
- Keep your knees slightly bent throughout the exercise to reduce strain on your joints.
- Focus on a full range of motion to fully engage and stretch the calf muscles.

Exercise: Seated Leg Curl

Target Muscles: Hamstrings (biceps femoris, semitendinosus, semimembranosus), calves (gastrocnemius)

Equipment: Leg Curl machine

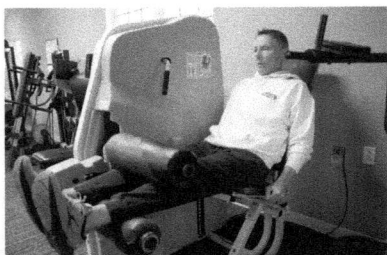

Starting Position   **Ending Position**

HOW TO DO THE EXERCISE:

1. Sit down on the leg curl machine. Keep your chest held high and your head up. Hook your legs under the leg curl bar. (See Starting Position)

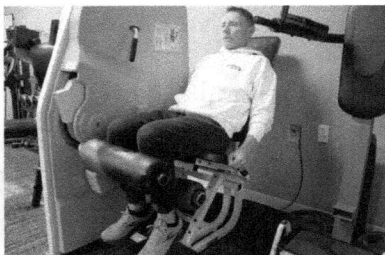

2. Slowly curl your heels toward your butt while simultaneously pressing your knees into the pads. This takes some practice to get used to. (See Ending Position)

3. Slowly return to the starting position. Only lower the weight for enough so the tension stays on the hamstrings. Your legs will not straighten out completely but they will get close.

Exercise Tip: *By squeezing the hamstrings in the contracted position, you increase the stress on the muscle.*

More Tips and Modifications:

- Avoid lifting your hips off the bench during the curl; learn to keep in contact with the seat.

- Ensure that your movements are slow and controlled to maximize muscle engagement and reduce the risk of injury.

- Adjust the machine's settings so that you can achieve a full range of motion without straining your knees.

Exercise: Leg Press

Target Muscles: Quadriceps, hamstrings, glutes, calves

Equipment: Leg Press machine

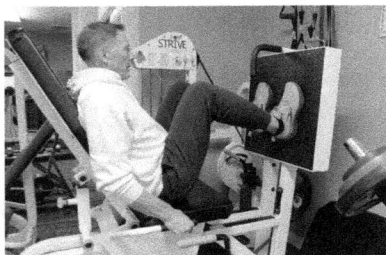

| **Starting Position** | **Ending Position** |

HOW TO DO THE EXERCISE:

1. Position yourself in the leg press machine making sure your butt and lower back against the pads. Your feet should be about shoulder-width apart on the platform. (See Starting Position)

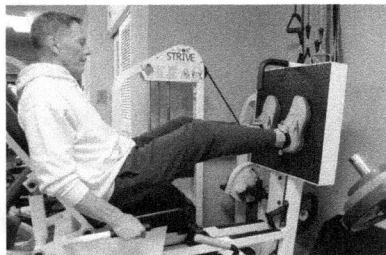

2. Push the weight up and release the handles. Lower the weight until you feel your thighs get close or touch your stomach. (See Ending Position)

3. Push through the heels, not through the toes. When you push through the heels, you will feel more quad and glute engagement.

Exercise Tip: *Your butt and lower back should always stay in contact with the bottom pads. If not, you put undue stress on the lower back. Also note the back pad of the leg press machine. Set the back up in an angled position, not in the flat position.*

More Tips and Modifications:

- Keep your feet flat on the platform throughout the entire range of motion.
- Keep your knees in line with your toes, avoiding any inward movement during the exercise.

Exercise: Leg Extension

Target Muscles: Quadriceps (rectus femoris, vastus lateralis, vastus medialis, vastus intermedius)

Equipment: Leg extension machine

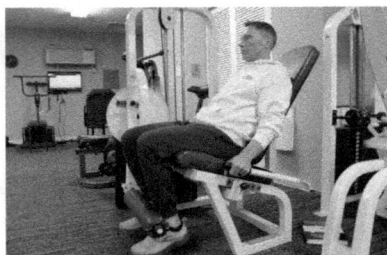

Starting Position

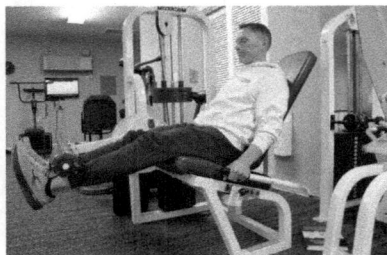

Ending Position

HOW TO DO THE EXERCISE:

1. Position yourself in the leg extension machine with your back flat against the backrest. Adjust the seat so that your knees align with the machine's pivot point, and your lower legs are positioned at about 90-degrees under the leg pads. (See Starting Position)

2. Slowly extend your feet into the pads. Make sure you feel the movement throughout the full extension. I like to squeeze my quads at the top of the movement. (See Ending Position)

Exercise Tip: *Maintain tension in your quadriceps throughout the movement, avoiding any sudden drops and make sure to use your quadriceps to move the weight and not momentum.*

More Tips and Modifications:

- Avoid swinging your legs or using momentum. The movement should be slow and controlled.

- Focus on squeezing your quads at the top of the movement for maximum activation.

Exercise: Lat Pulldown

Target Muscles: Latissimus dorsi (lats), biceps, shoulders (rear deltoids), and middle back (rhomboids, trapezius)

Equipment: Lat pulldown machine

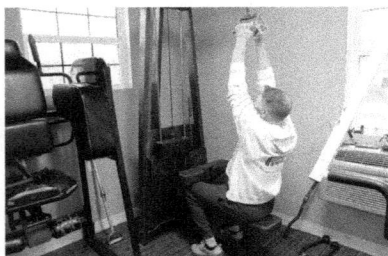

Starting Position   **Ending Position**

HOW TO DO THE EXERCISE:

1. Sit in front of the Pulldown machine making sure your legs are supported under the pads. Grab the bar and lean back slightly. (See Starting Position)

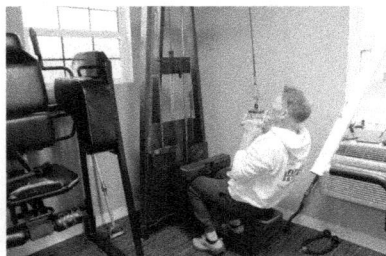

2. Bring the bar down to your sternum while simultaneously arching your back and pushing your chest up to meet the bar. (See Ending Position)

3. Return the bar slowly to close to the starting position and continue with your set.

Exercise Tip: *One of the most important points for back movements is to get the right "feel" for the movement. The ideal for proper back exercise is getting the back muscles to do the pulling and not the arm* *muscles. One of the ways that I have been able to get the proper feel for my lat muscles is to imagine the resistance against that back of your arms near your elbows. Next, I imagine trying to elbow someone behind me.*

More Tips and Modifications:

- Eliminate momentum when you pull the bar down; the movement should be controlled and initiated by the muscles in your back.

- Do not allow the bar to return to the top without control; the return movement should be smooth and steady.

- Keep your body more upright throughout the exercise to keep your lats engaged. Slightly leaning back is fine, but excessive leaning can reduce the effectiveness of the exercise.

Exercise: Chest Press

Target Muscles: Pectorals (chest muscles), triceps, anterior deltoids (front shoulders)

Equipment: Chest Press machine

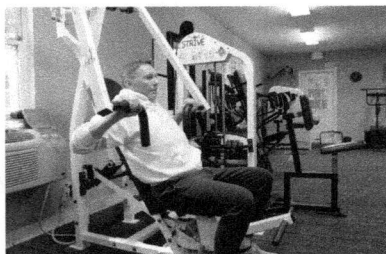

Starting Position   **Ending Position**

HOW TO DO THE EXERCISE:

1. Position yourself in the machine. Put your hands in the position where your palms are facing the ground. Keep your body in a position where your back and head is flat against the bench. Push against the handles until the arms are about fully extended but not locked out. (See Starting Position)

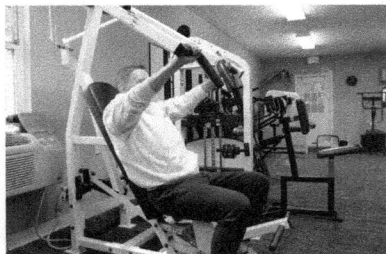

2. Slowly lower the handles until you feel a good stretch in your chest. (See Ending Position)

3. Push handles forward returning to starting position.

Exercise Tip: *Most machines keep you doing the exercises correctly, which is why I like to use them. However, the common mistake is to* *"squirm" or move around when the movement becomes difficult. Be careful not to fall into this pattern as soft tissue injury can occur.*

More Tips and Modifications:

- Keep your back pressed against the back pad throughout the movement. This will keep your back safe.
- Avoid Excessive elbow flaring, as this can place unnecessary stress on your shoulders. I let my elbows follow a natural line when I lower the weight.

Exercise: Seated Row

Target Muscles: Upper back, biceps, and rear deltoids

Equipment: Seated Row Machine

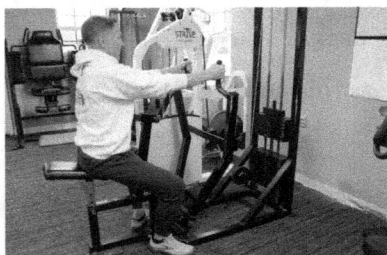

| Starting Position | Ending Position |

HOW TO DO THE EXERCISE:

1. Sit on the seated row machine facing forward. Grab the bar and lean back slightly. Use a neutral grip (palms facing each other) with your arms extended. (See Starting Position)

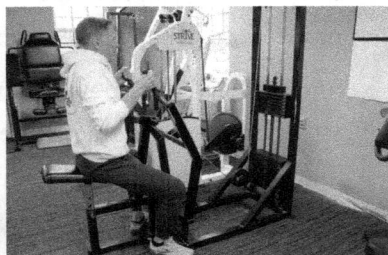

2. Slowly bring the bar towards your chest while simultaneously keeping your torso upright. (See Ending Position)

3. Return the bar slowly to close to the starting position and continue with your set.

Exercise Tip: *When you get into the contracted position, intentionally squeeze the muscle of the upper back together. The idea for proper back exercise is getting the back muscles to do the pulling and not the arm muscles.*

More Tips and Modification:

- Keep your back slightly arched and your chest lifted high throughout the entire range of motion.
- Make sure the movement is controlled and driven by your back muscles.

Exercise: Overhead Press

Target Muscles: Deltoids (shoulders), triceps, upper chest (pectorals), trapezius

Equipment: Overhead press machine (also known as shoulder press machine)

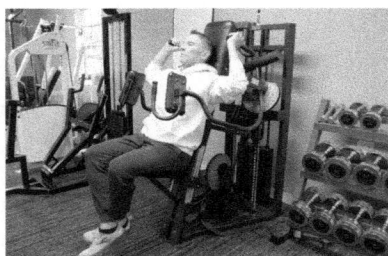

Starting Position   **Ending Position**

HOW TO DO THE EXERCISE:

1. Position yourself on the seat with your back flat against the bench and your hands firmly grasping the machine handles. (See Starting Position)

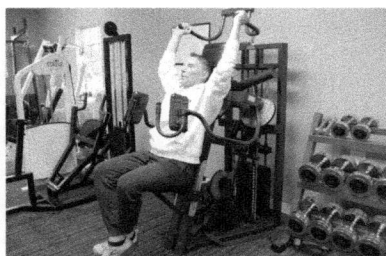

2. Slowly press the bar straight over your head, keeping your back flat against the bench. (See Ending Position)

3. Slowly return to the starting position.

Exercise Tip: *The most important aspect of this movement is to keep your back flat against the bench. Some people have the tendency when the weight gets heavier, to arch their back off the bench and squirm which can result in injury.*

More Tips and Modifications:

- Controlled Movement: Never use momentum when lifting the weight to reduce the risk of injury.
- Avoid Overextension: Keep your back in contact with the pad during the press. This reduces the chance for a lower back strain and increases the effectiveness of the exercise.

Exercise: Bicep Curl

Target Muscles: Biceps (biceps brachii)

Equipment: Bicep curl machine

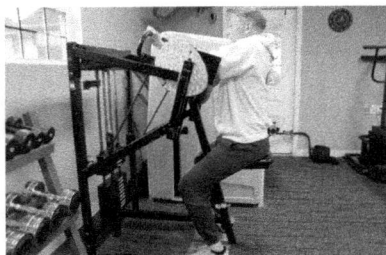

Starting Position   **Ending Position**

Note: The curl machine is very common in gyms, just find one that you feel comfortable with.

HOW TO DO THE EXERCISE:

1. Adjust the height of the machine seat so when you sit your shoulders are slightly (about 1-2 inches) higher than your hands. Keep your arm slightly bent. (See Starting Position)

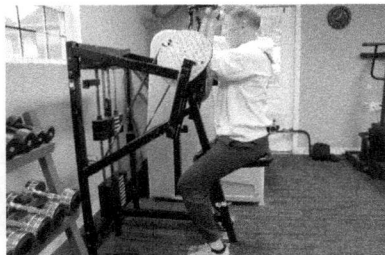

2. Slowly curl handles toward you feeling the tension throughout the whole movement. Bring your arms as far toward you as you can and flex the biceps hard at the top of the movement. (See Ending Position)

3. Slowly lower the weight into the starting position.

Exercise Tip: *The top part of the movement can give you a good contraction if you consciously squeeze hard at the top of the movement.*

When you lower the weight do not straighten your arms completely. This keeps undue stress off the elbow joints.

More Tips and Modifications:

- Controlled Contraction: When you get to the top of the movement, intentionally contract the biceps to increase the intensity of the exercise.
- Do Not Overextend: Do not over extend your elbows at the bottom of the movement. This will protect your joints.

Exercise: Tricep Pressdown

Target Muscles: Triceps (triceps brachii)

Equipment: Cable machine with a straight bar, rope, or V-bar attachment

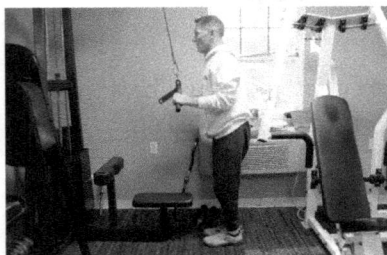

Starting Position   **Ending Position**

HOW TO DO THE EXERCISE:

1. Stand away from the Press down machine holding the bar in front of you so the cable is angling slightly away from you. Your elbows should be at your sides. (See Starting Position)

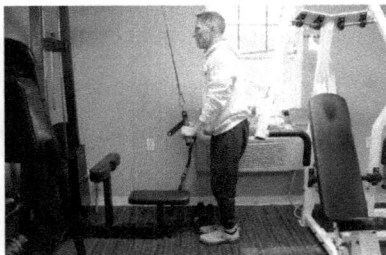

2. Slowly press the bar down and flex the triceps hard at the bottom of the movement. (See Ending Position)

3. Slowly return the bar to the starting position.

Exercise Tip: *When you are pressing the bar down, it should not go straight down but should arc a little away from your body. If you feel the most tension about two thirds of the way down, you are doing the movement optimally.*

More Tips and Modifications:

- Your elbows will want to flair out away from your body during the movement. Do your best to keep the elbows close to your sides.

- Moderate weight loads are best with this exercise. If you go too heavy, you lose the feel of the movement.

Exercise: Inverted Row

Target Muscles: Upper back (latissimus dorsi, rhomboids, trapezius), biceps, rear deltoids (back of shoulders), and core

Equipment: Smith machine, barbell in a squat rack, or suspension trainer (e.g., TRX)

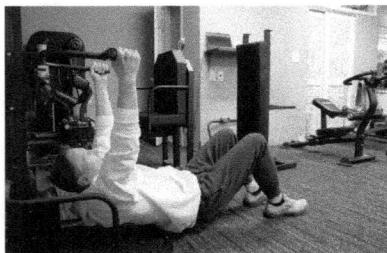

Starting Position   **Ending Position**

HOW TO DO THE EXERCISE:

1. Set a barbell in a squat rack or Smith machine at about waist height. Alternatively, you can use a suspension trainer. Position yourself under the bar so that your chest is directly underneath it. Your body should be in a straight line from head to heels, with your heels on the ground and your legs extended. (See Starting Position)

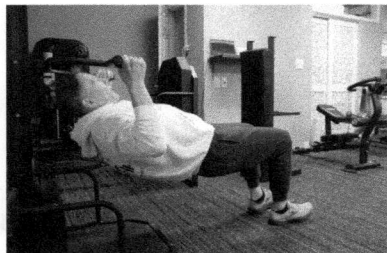

2. Slowly and deliberately pull your body up as high as you can. Intentionally flex the upper back by pulling the scapular together at the top of the movement. (See Ending Position)

3. Slowly return the bar to the starting position.

Exercise Tip: *When you are pulling your body up toward the top, make sure you squeeze the upper back muscles together. .*

More Tips and Modifications:

- **Body Alignment:** Keep your body in a straight line throughout the exercise.

- **Grip Variation:** You can vary your grip (overhand, underhand, or neutral) to target different muscles and add variety to the exercise.

- **Control the Movement:** Avoid using momentum to pull yourself up. Focus on a slow and controlled movement to maximize muscle engagement and effectiveness.

THE GOSPEL OF FITNESS

Exercise: Push-Up

Target Muscles: Chest (pectorals), shoulders (deltoids), triceps, core, and lower back

Equipment: None (bodyweight exercise)

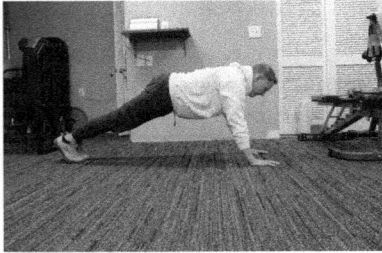

Starting Position   **Ending Position**

HOW TO DO THE EXERCISE:

1. Start with your arms straight, hands about shoulder with apart, feet hip width apart, palms and toes on the floor, and your body as straight as possible. (See Starting Position)

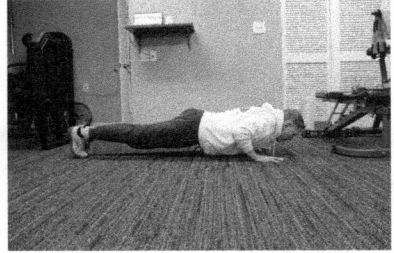

2. Lower your body slowly until you are almost touching the floor. (See See Ending Position)

3. Push yourself up slowly to the starting position but stop before complete lockout.

Exercise Tip: *If the exercise is too difficult with the form described above, put your knees on the floor to make the workout more manageable. Then try to keep your hips back and over your feet. This reduces* *tension on the upper body. As you get stronger, you can move your hips forward which increases the intensity of the exercise.*

More Tips and Modifications:

- Elbow Position: Keep your elbows at a 45-degree angle from your body to protect your shoulders and maximize chest engagement.

The Initial Fat Loss Plan

"Like holding your breath, dieting is against nature and nature will always win." – George Mateljan

With that said, I'm going to give you a plan.

Here's why I'm doing it: When you're starting out, you need a guide. That's so important.

In my experience as a trainer, some people can figure it out on their own but others need more specifics.

But stop and think about what I'm going to say here.

Most people fail for two reasons.

The first reason is they want to lose fat too fast.

The second reason is the diet is too restrictive.

I want you to start with this plan if you need to and stay on it for as long as you need. From there, I want you to branch out based on your goals.

When I say branching out, I want you to explore more foods and more recipes.

Over and over, I hear people say, "I really want to lose weight!" I understand what they are saying because weighing too much is obviously a problem. However, weight loss is not exactly what you are after.

You are pursuing **FAT LOSS!!**

Losing weight can be a combination of fat and muscle and muscle loss is very unhealthy. So our goal should be to drop body fat while maintaining, or in some cases, even building muscle. That's where High Intensity Training Comes in.

There are some very specific ways to do this. We use an approach that works as long as it's adhered to.

Most people think exercise is primary to losing body fat but this isn't necessarily true or at least it's not the whole picture.

Food intake is the key to losing body fat. Exercise figures in as it prevents muscle loss and increases metabolic condition.

The diet outline provided is based on caloric intake reduction or simply put: calories in, calories out.

There's more to it than that but if fat loss is the goal, you want to create a caloric-deficit, meaning you use more than you take in. You must understand that body fat is simply stored energy or calories. So to reduce the fat, the calorie intake must be reduced. This is a fact that cannot be changed!!

The general recommendation for FAT LOSS is about 1,400-1,700 per day for men and 1,100-1,400 per day for women. You can adjust the levels based on your personal responses but men should never drop below 1,200 or women below 1,000 unless under the advice of a trained medical professional.

If you want to find out how many calories you need per day, there's a simple way to do so. Multiply your current body weight by 12 if you're sedentary or by 15 if you're moderately active. This will give you your maintenance calorie amount.

I weigh 170 pounds. 170 times 15 is 2,550, and 170 times 12 is 2,040.

For fat loss, we want to reduce calories by 500–750 per day. I've done this for a while, and I know my maintenance calorie count is 2,300 per day. So, if I want to drop some fat, I'd reduce my calories by about 500–750 per day. That reduction puts me at about 1,550–1,800 calories for fat loss.

The following guidelines are just that—guidelines. You can swap out foods to suit your preferences, but make sure the calorie levels remain consistent.

I've provided several options to choose from while keeping things as simple as possible. This aligns with my Flexitarian approach. I'll give you several options and also show you how to incorporate daily fasts into your program.

Calorie-Controlled Meal Plan:

Breakfast: (Goal is approximately 300 calories)

- 1 egg cooked in a non-stick skillet (70 cal)
- ½ dry measure old fashioned oats (150 cal)
- 1 banana (100 cal)

Or

- 2 eggs (140 cal)
- 2 pieces of whole grain toast (140 cal)
- ½ cup cantaloupe (25 cal)

Or

- Meal replacement protein shake (300 cal)
- I use protein powder with almond milk

Or

Breakfast Protein Parfait (260 cal)

- 1/4 cup Greek yogurt, plain, fat-free
- 1/4 cup low-fat cottage cheese
- 1 scoop high-quality strawberry or vanilla protein powder
- 1/4 cup fresh berries
- 1 tablespoon pecan pieces, toasted

Here's what you need:

1. In a small bowl, use a whisk to combine the yogurt, cottage cheese, and protein powder.

Mix until well incorporated.

2. Place half of the yogurt mixture into a clear cup, top with the berries and then the remaining yogurt mixture. Top with pecans.

Snack: Goal is 100 calories for women, 200 for men—men can choose two.

Choose:

- Pack of nuts of your liking—I like almonds and cashews (100 cal)
- 1 apple (100 cal)
- 2 cups popcorn (100 cal)—I use the skinny pop brand

Lunch: (Goal is approximately 300 calories)

- 2 slices whole grain bread (140 cal)
- Lettuce and tomato (30 cal)
- 2 ounces nitrate free lunch meat (70 cal)
- 1 apple (100)

Or

- 2 slices whole-grain bread (140 cal)
- 1 banana (80 cal)
- 1 tablespoon almond butter (98 cal)

Dinner: Goal is 300-400 calories

- 1 cup brown rice (216 cal)
- ½ cup black beans (114 cal)
- ¼ cup fresh salsa (50 cal)

Recipe for fresh salsa:

- 2 small fresh tomatoes
- 1/2 medium red onion
- 2 serrano or 1 jalapeño pepper, stems, ribs, and seeds removed (less or more to taste)
- 1/2 cup chopped cilantro
- Salt and freshly ground black pepper to taste
- 1 pinch dried oregano, or more to taste

Chop all ingredients and mix together. Chill in the fridge.

Or

- Any healthy frozen dinner (300 cal)
- 2 slices bread (70 cal)

Or

- Large salad with variety of veggies with light dressing (150 cal)
- Lettuce, broccoli, mushrooms, tomatoes and onions. These are very low in calories so make it big!
- 1 chicken breast (150 cal)

Dinner is where you're welcome to start experimenting with different recipes. Here's a good one:

Potatoes, Corn and, Salmon

- 1 potato (100 cal)
- 1 sweetcorn cob (75 cal)
- 1 skinless salmon filet (150 cal)
- 1 medium tomato (30 cal)

For the dressing:

- 1 tbsp red wine vinegar
- 1 tbsp extra-virgin olive oil
- Chopped onions

Sprinkle basil leaves.

Boil potatoes in water until tender, adding corn for last 5 minutes.

Bake salmon with seasoning of your choice

Veggie Wrap (360 cal)

- 1 wheat, spinach, or whole-grain tortilla
- 1/4 cup hummus
- Chopped lettuce
- 2 tablespoons nuts
- Chopped red peppers
- Shredded carrots
- Shredded cabbage

Steps:

Wrap all ingredients in the tortilla and roll it up.

Optional Snack: Goal is 100 calories for women, 200 for men — so men choose two.

Choose:

- Pack of nuts of your liking (100 cal)
- 1 apple (100 cal)
- 2 cups popcorn (100 cal)

Or choose from dinner menu options in recipes section.

You must measure food and count calories!!! I based this calorie count at 1,500-1,800/day for fat loss for men and 1,100-1,500 per day for fat loss for women!

This program can get you started. You can follow it exactly or adjust it to fit you.

Here's an alternative eating plan that I use. It's Intermittent Fasting. Let's talk about it.

Intermittent Fasting Works

"Fasting is the single greatest natural healing therapy. It is nature's ancient, universal 'remedy' for many problems."
– Elson Haas, M.D..

If there is any one thing that's changed my life, it's fasting.

I don't fast for days, although I've done some overnight fasts. I simply fast for hours.

As a competitive bodybuilder, I was obsessed with the ideas of muscle building and fat loss.

This led to some very strict dieting with one day per week of being off my diet. This one day per week led to some incredible binge eating. I literally ate over 10,000 calories on one particular binge day. I remember in my journal the day started off with this entry:

"½ cheesecake"

Then there was all kinds of other entries and then this entry:

"The other ½ cheesecake"

Basically, I had an eating disorder. I'd diet down and gain the weight back, over and over again.

This went on for many years. I'd pray for release from what I'd call "Food Bondage." I describe this as an obsession with food. What am I going to eat next? What's my weight? My body fat percentage? How do I look? And on and on it went.

After many years of this, I read something about intermittent fasting and because I tried EVERYTHING else, I figured why not try this?

I started fasting until 5-6 pm on Mondays and Thursdays and I loved it! It was a breakthrough.

I just noticed how good I felt on those days and how food even tasted better. I still had to be aware of binging but I was gaining some traction.

Then I read a post about a guy who did daily fasts, and his thought was, "If I feel this good when I fast, why not make it my daily routine?"

That made sense to me, so I tried it and I've never looked back.

Here are some of the benefits of Intermittent Fasting:

- **Helps lose/maintain weight**
- **Improves metabolic health**
- **Reduces inflammation**
- **Increases lifespan**

- **Improves cognitive health**
- **Helps with insulin sensitivity**
- **Has cardiovascular benefits**

"Everyone who does intermittent fasting talks about it as a lifestyle, not a diet. They come for weight loss, but stay for the health benefits."
– Author Unknown

The Ideal Lifestyle Eating Plan

I've lost fat and kept it off by making a lifestyle change - Me

I'd really love for you to adopt a style of eating that will help you lose fat and keep it off. I started you with a regular routine of eating, now we branch out.

You have to find what fits you, but as I showed you previously, I switched to more fruits and vegetables, grains, and lower fat high-fiber foods.

This allows me to eat foods that taste great yet I feel full and I'm not yo yo dieting anymore.

If I were to summarize it:

My eating style is flexible with foods I actually enjoy

- **Starchy vegetables such as sweet potatoes, squash, and peas.**

- **Fruits such as berries, apples, grapes, oranges, peaches, figs, bananas, and kiwi.**
- **Whole grains such as oatmeal, buckwheat, quinoa, and rice.**
- **Legumes such as chickpeas, beans, and lentils.**
- **Almond and coconut milk**
- **Protein powders**
- **Nuts and seeds**
- **Both lean and fatty meats**
- **And some junk food every now and then but not too often**

I'm still free to eat whatever I want and change as needed.

Here's what one of my days can look like:

Wake up early and have some black coffee. I generally have two cups.

On days I workout, I'll do the machine-based plan, or a variation of it, that I have in the workout session of this book.

On days I go to the gym to train clients, I'll have my protein shake at 1:45. I usually wait to eat until 3:00-3:30, but my schedule will force me to change times.

Protein shake

- 1 ½ cup almond milk (60 calories)
- 1 frozen banana and 1 to 1 1/2 cup frozen mangos (200 cal)

- 2 scoops protein - I use muscle tech or Jen's dairy free protein (280 calories 40-50 grams of protein or a Ka'Chava meal replacement)

Total of 540 calories

I'll take a green drink with me and drink that later, maybe 3:30 - 4:00, and I'll also take my fiber drink then.

When I come home at 5:00, I will have what Jen cooked for dinner. One meal she makes that I like is vegetable chili. I will have it in a tortilla wrap and put some brown rice with it. It will be a large amount of food and it'll be filling. I'll have a few nuts after that.

- Brown rice approximately 2 cups (400 cal)
- Vegetarian chili 2 cups (400 cal)
- Wrap (70 cal)

Total 870 calories

I'll usually have some popcorn which is 40 calories per cup and some nuts

This will be about 250 calories

I'll walk on the treadmill immediately after.

If I'm hungry later, I'll have an apple or a banana.

Which is another 100 calories.

That'll be pretty much it.

I'll get about 70-100 grams of protein and about 1,700-1,800 calories per day.

My weight remains very stable, I feel great, I enjoy my food, and I'm never starving myself.

I have a list of go-to foods that I enjoy from local restaurants and they're very healthy options. Or I'll eat what Jen makes as she's a great cook.

If you notice, I don't eat much meat. If I want it, I'll eat it, but I feel so good with what I'm doing now and I've been doing this for well over a year now, I just don't see any reason to change.

I'm simply free to eat what I like and I enjoy it and I'm no longer in bondage to food!

And I underlined that for a reason.

A lot of people can relate to that "bondage to food" part.

I will tell you it's very freeing to not have to deal with that any longer!

And I no longer count calories! I've gotten good at "intuitive" eating.

Tips For Intermittent Fasting

How do I start? What do I eat?

Let's go through the days of the first week:

Monday

Breakfast is some water and/or a cup of black coffee (no cream or sugar) or a cup of tea.

We are going to have lunch and dinner today.

As a side note, as long as you're healthy, you'll be ok and you'll make it to lunch. Some people might just completely get scared and think their blood sugar is going to fall through the floor.

This most likely isn't going to happen. If you struggle with the psychology of not having breakfast, just take the approach of having to fast for a blood test at the doctor's office. You'll get to eat, you just have to wait for a little while.

Lunch – have a meal. Something healthy if possible, a fresh organic salad is best if possible. If not, simply eat what is in front of you and stop eating before you're stuffed. This could be 11:00 or noon. Whatever is open, don't just eat because it's time to eat, wait for hunger.

I know some people need actual answers to the question, 'What do I eat?' If a salad isn't an option for you, here's a possible lunch:

Lunchmeat Sandwich: 2 slices of healthy bread, lettuce, tomato, organic cage-free chicken breast, mustard or mayo, and cheese. Add an apple and water or tea.

As the day goes on, you might have more water, coffee, or tea in the afternoon. Avoid snacking altogether.

Dinner could be around 6:00 or 7:00. Simply focus on having good food. If someone cooks dinner, eat what's in front of you, but don't have seconds.

As you go through this process, you'll likely fail at times or fall off the wagon. But here's the thing.

THERE IS NO FAILURE WITH THIS LIFESTYLE.

If you overeat, simply take a break before your next meal.

There are times when you might just have dinner and do a full day of no food.

Experiment and see what works for you. You are the scientist here. Learn to understand feedback.

So here's what your week can look like:

Monday: Fast until noon. As you get accustomed to fasting you can go longer.

Tuesday and Wednesday: Go with my "Eat Regular Today."

Thursday: This is a fasting day. Maybe you can go a little longer with the fast.

Friday - Saturday - Sunday: "Eat Regular Today."

When I say "Eat Regular Today," that could be just breakfast/lunch/dinner for you. Whatever is considered "regular" for you. Just don't overeat!!

THIS IS JUST AN EXAMPLE!

The beauty of fasting or eating less food is the freedom it creates.

For example, if you're going to go to dinner with some friends, you can do an all-day fast or eat a light lunch and then really enjoy dinner! I do this all the time!

Once again, learn to experiment! Be smart; play it safe but learn your body!

Let me give you some basics once again:

Take your time with fasting.

I don't want you to go and just start skipping meals without a plan. Try not having breakfast one day and note how you feel. Keep experimenting and find what works best for you.

Eat quality food.

There are times when you won't have a choice and you'll have to eat what's in front of you. That's ok. Just don't do that every day! Follow the 80/20 rule. Try to eat clean, healthy foods 80% of the time.

Don't over fast.

Learn to experiment and find what works for you. This is not about starving yourself; it's about learning to control appetite and eating less food, less often but also eating quality food.

Create a lifestyle.

If you can't do it for the rest of your life, then don't do it at all. Don't restrict and torture yourself. You can't diet forever; it simply doesn't work. However, if you can learn to find something you can live healthy with then you're on your way.

It's not for everyone.

Fasting might not work for you. Try it and see. If you're pregnant, nursing, hypoglycemic, diabetic, or have any history of health problems, you shouldn't do it. Consult your physician before trying anything like this. Give it an honest chance though; it works for most people!

Use common sense.

Here's a common sense approach:

- Eat quality food
- Eat slower
- Listen to your body. If you're really hungry, then eat.
- Control portions
- Don't binge when you break the fast.

I'll be the first to admit I've done this! Fasting is not an excuse for binge eating. You still have to count calories. You still have to weigh yourself. You still have to DRINK PLENTY OF WATER. Fasting is simply a way to control the amount of food you're eating!

The Fasting Mindset

Let's look at that first day of fasting. Think of it like preparing to get your blood drawn.

Imagine your doctor says, 'We're going to need a blood sample. I don't want you to eat or drink anything that has calories until we get that sample.' During the fast, you can have as much water as you want, as well as black coffee or tea. Avoid diet soda—it's just not good for you.

Set a time for your fast to begin and end. It can start early to help you ease into it or later in the day, depending on what works best for you. It takes time for your body to adjust, but it will adapt.

When I started fasting, I always broke my fast with an apple. Then, I'd wait about 30 minutes to an hour before having dinner. I also made sure to stay within my calorie range.

When you break your fast, eat real food—no processed or fast food. Treat your body well.

Fast again on Thursday. Repeat this process for a few weeks.

You can incorporate fasting into the above diet plan if you'd like. It will require discipline, and you might feel a bit uncomfortable at first, but your body will adjust.

Extra Tips For Fat Loss

Walk for 30 minutes after your evening meal.

Just a leisurely walk; you don't need to overstress your body.

If the evening doesn't work, adjust your walk to fit you. Remember, I'm giving you guidelines not laws.

Drink cold water.

I will admit I'm not great at this but it really does help and it causes your body to burn extra calories by having to heat the water up.

Get extra sleep when you can.

Getting enough sleep may help prevent increases in calorie intake and appetite that can happen when you're sleep deprived.

Those of us who don't get enough sleep have an increased appetite and generally eat more calories.

This sleep tip could actually change your life and help your health in incredible ways.

You lose fat when you sleep.

Learn to control stress levels.

Stress releases cortisol and cortisol isn't conducive to fat loss.

Sleep

I think sleep was my problem in school. If school had started at 4 in the afternoon, I'd be a college graduate today.
- George Foreman, former heavyweight boxer.

According to an article in the premiere issue of the NFPT Review, sleep is critically important. They write:

"One of the most inherent values of sleep is the concurrent breakdown of toxins in the cerebrospinal fluid that accumulate during waking hours. After 48 hours of sleep deprivation, test subjects have been found to display significant long- and short-term memory loss, as well as a reduction in their ability to reason and communicate effectively.

All of these symptoms have been attributed, in part, to the buildup of toxins in the cerebrospinal fluid during waking hours. It is also interesting to note that the rate of toxin buildup in the cerebrospinal fluid is unique to each individual, thus explaining why some people can function effectively on less sleep than others."

What exactly does this mean for us? One thing it means is that we need to get enough sleep. In our society, we are pushed to the limits of our abilities on a daily basis. We're encouraged to work more hours and get less rest in order to "make ends meet."

This mentality, however, causes us to function at much lower levels than we're capable of. Based on the quote above, if I don't get enough sleep, I won't function anywhere near my full potential.

If I reduce my sleep by just one hour per night and the toxin buildup in my cerebrospinal fluid isn't completely removed, it will accumulate. Over time, this buildup can reach levels that lead to short-term memory loss, poor communication skills, and a reduced ability to reason. That's not how I want to function in my personal or professional life.

Sleep also restores our body's energy supplies that are depleted throughout the day. The amount of sleep required varies from person to person, depending on the type and intensity of work they do. For example, someone who does physically demanding labor will need more sleep than someone whose work is primarily mental.

Teenagers, due to the hormonal changes in their bodies, require significantly more sleep than they did as children.

There are people who have trouble sleeping. This can include inability to fall asleep or stay sleeping for more than a few hours.

Before and After Pictures

When a client comes and they're motivated to get some results, I suggest taking a before picture, and at the end of eight weeks, to take an after picture.

This is just a suggestion but it does help with motivation.

Here's how to do it:

You want to standardize the before and after, meaning you want to take the pictures under the same condition, with the same clothes on. I'm not a fan of cut offs or tank tops, just some everyday, walking around clothes.

To standardize make sure:

- **The lighting is consistent.**
- **The distance of both photos are consistent.**
- **The poses are the same. Just a relaxed front and side pose will suffice.**
- **The time of day is consistent.**

This will give you a "true look" when it comes to your results.

Remember this is just a suggestion as some people would rather not do these, however, they are a great motivator.

Once you've completed them, post your results and send them over to me at Steve@fitnessandmore.net. I'll feature them on my website: www.fitnessandmore.net.

Questions and Answers

"You want answers?" "I want the truth!"
Lieutenant Daniel Kaffee and Colonel Nathan Jessep,
A Few Good Men

I like to run; can I run on this program?

I don't suggest running, especially as we get older. I've had many referrals from local health practitioners for injuries related to running. The idea of walking after meals is to aid in digestion and slightly increase body temperature.

Choosing to run will disrupt digestion and upset your stomach and it will increase the chance of running-related joint issues. I'm really not a fan of long distance running but I do some sprinting as I like it and it doesn't hurt my body.

What about ketogenic diets?

I've used ketogenic diets before and I've done fine with them. The major problem with the ketogenic diet is underemphasizing calories and overemphasizing carbohydrates.

I've seen people go on ketogenic diets and eat copious amounts of proteins and fats and they will actually lose weight quickly but the weight loss has more to do with water loss than fat loss.

Fat loss takes time and calories matter for fat loss, so if you choose a ketogenic diet, eat real food and count calories. This will make sure you're losing fat.

What about fat burning supplements?

Fat burning supplements will work for a while and then they stop when your body adapts to them. Your body wants to stay in what's called homeostasis, which simply means it wants to remain as is and it doesn't really want to change, so you have to learn to coax it and not force it.

I don't recommend fat burners as a way of life, nor would I even suggest using them at all as some fat burners have major side effects.

I do remember one of the strongest fat burners I've ever used. It was called "Ultimate Orange," and it was strong! Drug-like strong! It was banned for a while but I'd never use anything like that again.

I like to do more cardio. How much should I do?

You don't need any more cardio than lifting and walking. Too much cardio creates undue stress and raises cortisol levels. When cortisol levels are high, fat loss diminishes and strength decreases.

What we're looking for in an exercise program is the least amount of exercise to elicit the best possible response. More exercise is not going to produce better results and in most cases will slow progress.

What's the best time of day to workout?

Experiment with the time of day you workout. I find that 9–10 AM is optimal for me. Others like to workout early as a good way to start the day. Some people like a later in the evening workout.

One more thought for busy people: Sometimes you just have to fit the workout into your schedule so your time of day can vary. Just workout when you have the time to do so, but make sure you fit it in.

I need to lose weight in my abs. What exercises should I do?

We do several different abs exercises in the program that will help strengthen the underlying ab muscles. However, you can do ab exercises literally all day long and you won't lose weight in the abs.

The reason is, you can't spot reduce. What that means is you can't lose fat in one area of your body by using exercise. When you reduce body fat as a whole, then and only then will you be able to see your abs.

If you go back to the watching your diet section of the book, you'll see that body fat is reduced by creating a calorie deficit within reason.

Can I continue on with the program after eight weeks?

Absolutely! I'd suggest taking one week off from training after the eight week program is over, as it will allow your system to recover, thereby setting you up for another good eight week run at the program.

Will my workouts help my mental health?

*100%! Workout regularly and **workout hard!** Walk daily and eat real food. This will really help your mental health and it fits in with my aging gracefully model.*

Controlling your mental health has various aspects to it but my 3-W Approach To Fitness works perfectly for mental health benefits.

I use a semaglutide for weight loss; is it safe for me to strength train?

It's not only safe, it's imperative that you strength train. These drugs help with weight loss but remember what we're after is FAT LOSS!

Semaglutide use causes fat loss, muscle loss, and bone loss. We only want fat loss and strength training helps prevent and or minimize muscle loss and bone loss.

What about other methods of training, such as hiking or bike riding?

I do other methods of training, i.e., Jiu-Jitsu, but I do it more because I really like it. It has community, it's fun, and it makes me feel good.

I would combine these other methods with the strength training plan that I laid out.

I do think it's good to challenge yourself in different areas. It's fine to go for a long hike or try different things, but just be aware of how your body responds to what you're doing.

Final Instructions: Putting It All Together

Let's make sure we have our gameplan down and we're ready to get this healthy lifestyle started. Here is a summary of our approach:

1 - Pick a start day. Mondays are usually best.

2 - Pick your diet plan. You can do the intermittent fasting, the calorie controlled plan, or combine the two. You will track calories on both plans but you want to find the plan that fits you best. It's fine to alternate the plans as long as you track your progress.

3 - Weigh in. You want to record your starting weight and ending weight on the same scale, just for consistency.

4 - Pick your program. You have the option of the home or gym workout. You can also combine the two. The whole idea of the program is to make it fit you—just be consistent with your workouts. Follow the workout plan as outlined but make adjustments if needed as you start to understand how your body responds to exercise.

5 - Prep your food. Go to the grocery store and get your food for the week.

6 - Drink plenty of water. Create a new habit of water drinking to help with fat loss. Cold water is best.

7- Walk 30 minutes per day. Try to walk for 30 minutes after your evening meal if possible. If it's not possible, simply walk when you can.

8 - Get extra sleep. Extra sleep is vitally important. I can't emphasize the importance of sleep enough. It'll help with muscle recovery and fat loss.

9 - Reduce stress. Stress releases cortisol which promotes fat gain and muscle loss. Less stress equals better results.

10 - Enjoy the process. You're going to look better, feel better and move better, enjoy it! This eight week process will require some discipline but it's worth it and it can actually be fun.

ENDNOTES

1 https://www.niddk.nih.gov/health-information/health-statistics/overweight-obesity#:~:text=Adults,-Age%2Dadjusted%20percentage&text=the%20above%20table-,Nearly%201%20in%203%20adults%20(30.7%25)%20are%20overweight.,obesity%20(including%20severe%20obesity).

2 https://my.clevelandclinic.org/health/diseases/22310-muscle-atrophy

3 https://www.ncbi.nlm.nih.gov/pmc/articles/PMC2804956/

4 https://www.ncbi.nlm.nih.gov/books/NBK560813/#:~:text=Sarcopenia%20is%20a%20musculoskeletal%20disease,system%20or%20impair%20physical%20activity.

5 https://pmc.ncbi.nlm.nih.gov/articles/PMC2804956/

6 https://www.cbass.com/Biomarkers.htm

7 https://familyfoodllc.com/halloween-candy-calories-and-what-it-takes-to-burn/

8 https://www.nia.nih.gov/health/falls-and-falls-prevention/older-adults-and-balance-problems

9 https://personaltrainertoday.com/what-said-says

10 https://urbanvybe.com/three-components-well-balanced-exercise-routine/#:~:text=The%20three%20components%20to%20a%20well%2Dbalanced%20exercise%20routine%20include,strength%20training%2C%20and%20flexibility%20training.

11 https://traineracademy.org/blog/personal-training-industry-statistics/#:~:text=According%20to%20the%20most%20recent,2.2%25%20growth%20in%20 2021%20alone.

12 Shilts MK, Horowitz M, Townsend MS. Goal setting as a strategy for dietary and physical activitybehavior change: A review of the literature. American Journal of Health Promotion. 2004;19(2):81–93. doi: 10.4278/0890-1171-19.2.81

13 https://www.builtstrength.com.au/diet/is-fitbit-calorie-burn-accurate-what-you-need-to-know/

14 https://www.abbott.com/corpnewsroom/nutrition-health-and-wellness/5-tips-for-taking-charge-of-your-health.html#:~:text=Take%20control%20of%20your%20health,activity%20are%20best%20for%20you.

15 https://selecthealth.org/blog/2019/02/why-weight-lifting-is-good-for-heart-health

16 https://www.sciencedirect.com/science/article/pii/S2095254624000498#:~:text=A%20single%20bout%20of%20exercise,to%2024%20h%20post%2Dexercise.

17 (https://www.sydney.edu.au/news-opinion/news/2020/02/11/strength-training-can-help-protect-the-brain-from-degeneration.html#:~:text=The%20long%2Dterm%20study%20found,role%20in%20learning%20and%20memory.)

18 https://www.workoutgarage.com/blog/inroadtheory

19 https://www.realsimple.com/health/fitness-exercise/walking-benefits

20 I went to Darden's home for a consultation and took notes of what he told me.

21 Dr. Robert Cywes M.D. Ph.D. #CarbAddictionDoc @DrCywesCarbAddictionDoc

22 Dr. Ellington Darden, Killing Fat, page 70 Rodale 2019

23 https://www.goodreads.com/book/show/198359.Beyond_the_120_Year_Diet

24 https://www.healthcentral.com/chronic-health/how-hunger-hormones-control-weight-loss

25 https://www.burnthefatblog.com/nutrition-professor-loses-27-pounds-on-twinkie-diet/

26 https://www.mayoclinic.org/healthy-lifestyle/nutrition-and-healthy-eating/in-depth/fiber/art-20043983

27 https://www.health.harvard.edu/press_releases/get-nutrients-from-food-not-supplements

28 https://www.health.harvard.edu/press_releases/get-nutrients-from-food-not-supplements

29 https://www.healthline.com/nutrition/7-health-benefits-of-water

30 NFPT Magazine, Dec/Jan Issue 1999, Page 1, Ron J. Clark Publisher, NFPT Research Group

31 https://pubmed.ncbi.nlm.nih.gov/20145778/

ABOUT THE AUTHOR

Steve McKinney, owner of Fitness and More, Inc.

Innovator of the 3-W Approach To Fitness

1st Class Personal Trainer, NFPT, for over 30 years

Post Rehab Training Specialist

1990 Mr. Southern Illinois Light Heavyweight and Overall Winner

1987 Top 5 Finisher, Mr. Midwest

Jiu-Jitsu Black Belt

2-Time IBJJF Pan Ams Silver Medalist

Pastor

Instagram: @fitnessandmorestl
Facebook: @stevemckinney
YouTube: @FitnessandMoreInc

www.ingramcontent.com/pod-product-compliance
Lightning Source LLC
Chambersburg PA
CBHW050649270326
41927CB00012B/2941